FIST PUMPS

The Prescription for Physician Burnout

(A Self-Help Book to Lift Up Physicians and Healthcare Providers Who Serve)

by Scott MacDiarmid, MD

Dedication

To my wife Andrea, who rescued me from myself twice. You led me to love Jesus Christ and motivated me to refuse to live in the valley of burnout. You and Lindsey are my mountaintop.

CONTENTS

FOREWORD

I met Scott in the operating room locker room. He seemed like a happy-go-lucky Canadian urologist who belonged in the sequel to *Strange Brew*. I didn't know he was a writer, or a nationally recognized academic leader in urology, or that he spends his spare time in lecture halls sharing his personal insights battling burnout with thousands of medical professionals across the nation. I certainly didn't know he was a deep thinker, or a "noticer," who studies the world and the people around him with an unshakable caring heart. Our collegial friendship grew over the years, but never anything beyond casual conversation.

Then one day Scott and I were in the operating room locker room, and I was shaken. I was broken. I was in the midst of managing a patient who was plagued with addiction—his legs were dying before our very eyes. I had poured my heart and soul into trying to help him, but all my best medical efforts had failed. He was lashing out at me with every ounce of venom he could muster, blaming and threatening me over how I had failed to save his leg. I was devastated, overcome with doubt, failure, and fear. I was drowning in the negativity that was pouring out of this patient's soul.

When I shared this with Scott, he reached out to me with a gentle, caring touch. "Let me send you a couple of chapters from a book I'm working on about burnout." After reading a couple of pages, I was hooked. He had a real story to tell. With a real purpose. Intended for real people. Coming from a real heart.

Over the next two years, I have had the blessing of tagging along with Scott as he has developed this book. I have learned about his history, his journey into the valley of burnout, and his personal path to the mountaintop. I have been able to begin my own healing process, fueled by his commitment, his thoughts, and the insights that he shares in this book. He inspires his fellow humans.

Scott will take you on a journey exploring the factors that may be impacting your ability to love your job and your professional life. He will teach you some real-world techniques to strengthen your suit of armor, to allow you to charge into your daily battles and create love in your daily professional life. He will help you find your path to the mountaintop. He will help you come to understand how critical you really are to those around you. He will help you remember your purpose. He will inspire you to become the inspiration for others. That's how this works.

Scott honored me with asking me to write this foreword. We have worked on this book together, struggling with the "voice," with structure, with rhythm, the audience, and with the message. He has honored me by allowing me to contribute some small passages that we have woven into the tapestry of his story. We are both excited to see our coffee-table creativity take life in print, and we hope that you find meaning and value in the message.

He always said, even if he was only ever able to help a single person with this book, then all the years of effort would have been worth it. Well, I'm no longer the same broken man I was in the operating room locker room. And I think the list of people that he is going to help is only just beginning.

The goal of this book is not to "fix" burnout. The goal of this book is to learn how to position yourself on the path to healing, to position yourself on the path to your mountaintop.

Enjoy the journey,

Joshua Landau, MD
Orthopedic Surgeon

Introduction

As a practicing urologist, I am excited to share with you *Fist Pumps: The Prescription for Physician Burnout.* It's the prescription to help the endless number of physicians and other healthcare providers who are suffering from burnout, who yearn to feel joyful and fulfilled when caring for patients.

The fist pump is a universal gesture of triumph or affirmation used by athletes and others that is both encouraging and uplifting. There's just something about it that makes you feel great.

Imagine yourself as a provider in clinic or walking out of the operating room with your forearm raised and fist clenched and doing a fist pump in celebration. And imagine you did this several times daily, regardless of your circumstances, and each fist pump was associated with thinking, feeling, verbalizing, or doing something positive. Wow, in today's healthcare system, wouldn't that be something?

In this book, you will learn that every decision, choice, declaration, and action that helps you fight burnout and find joy is the prescription for your success. And that you can give yourself a congratulatory fist pump for each one. The gesture will affirm, encourage, and propagate your healthy thoughts, feelings, words, and behaviors, and it will become the symbol of your self-prescribed treatment. Taking personal responsibility and helping yourself is rewarded with a fist pump. It is the prescription for burnout.

Physician burnout is a big deal. It's a big deal to those suffering from it, to their patients, to those around them, to the healthcare system, and to the nation. The over-corporatization of the American healthcare system, which has fueled the fire that is burning out physicians and other providers, represents

1

one of the most important societal issues of our time.

Like many physicians, I have given my life to the practice of medicine and to helping others. It's an all-in commitment, perhaps a way of life. For the most part I have been successful with my career, my family, my friends and community, my standard of living. For decades, my shoulders were straightened by my success, pride, dedication, and sacrifice.

But more recently, I began struggling, realizing I no longer enjoyed practicing medicine like I used to. I became frustrated and short-tempered. I was easily angered, bitter, and resentful. My actions and behavior began affecting important relationships with friends, and even family.

I also noticed other physicians with their shoulders slumped, their faces prematurely aged by stress and loss of hope. Others appear fearful or too busy and overwhelmed to even realize that they are not happy or fulfilled. Early retirements, with a "just get me to the finish line" attitude and a mindset of "do I have to do this for thirty more years?" have become a new norm. Yes, burnout is insidious and destructive.

In my own battle with burnout, I learned many helpful thoughts and strategies that I want to share with others. Practicing in Canada, New Zealand, England, and now in the U.S. in both academic and private practice has given me unique perspectives and experiences that have helped me and I believe will be beneficial to you as well.

Since recognizing this issue of burnout in myself and colleagues, I came to realize that my goal—an ambitious one—is to lift up physicians and healthcare providers who serve. I want to create a world that nourishes healthcare providers and brings them happiness and meaning when caring for patients. A world that enables and encourages them to live out their purpose of using their gifts and talents to help others. A world in which burnout is rare, and better still, non-existent. Yes, this is a lofty goal, but with millions of like-minded people, we can speak up as one and benefit all.

About the Book

I'm inviting physicians, nurses, advanced practice providers, and the millions of young men and women aspiring to be healthcare providers to join our journey to fight burnout and to find joy when caring for patients and our nation.

Fist Pumps is divided into four parts. Some sections are intentionally detailed and pragmatic, while others are more inspirational and thought-provoking. I encourage you to push through each chapter, recognizing at times you may feel overwhelmed or fatigued doing the work of digging deeply into your career and your life. The battle against burnout is difficult, but perseverance will reward many.

Part 1, The Crisis, identifies and sounds the alarm that **we have a healthcare crisis . . . and the crisis is now**. Healthcare costs are soaring out of control, quality is deteriorating, and physicians are burning out and checking out in record numbers. Living in the valley of burnout can be devastating, and its causes are multifactorial. A deep understanding of its etiologies and how it affects each individual is an important step in their battle against burnout.

Part 2, Successful Battle Strategies in the Fight Against Burnout, discusses strategies that will help equip physicians to fight burnout and find joy. It details solutions and survival tactics that will help make you a great warrior, allowing you to ascend out of the valley of burnout and reach your mountaintop of happiness and fulfillment. The mountaintop is where you find meaning and live out your purpose. It's that meaningful place in life where you realize that all the negatives and stresses associated with the practice of medicine are worth it.

Part 3, Effectively Managing the Greed Virus, provides additional solutions and survival tactics that will enable you to manage the rapidly spreading greed virus that is killing healthcare and promoting burnout. The seven systems of the body of healthcare include the patients, the physicians and other providers, hospitals, third-party payers, the manufacturers of drugs and equipment, the legal profession, and the government. Each one has been infected with greed, entitlement, and unrealistic expectations, which in turn is stressing providers and promoting burnout. Like most viruses, it cannot be eradicated but it can be effectively managed. While part 2 offers important mindset advice, part 3 provides practical steps to deal with the stressors within each of the seven systems, including those that are self-inflicted.

In part 4, Finishing Strong, we reflect and discuss numerous ways of thinking that help produce healthy emotions, words, actions, and a meaningful life. We will face many of the fears that are pulling us down into the valley of burnout and emphasize that serving others in all five life domains—work, family, friends, community, and personal health—is the ultimate key to success.

I have invited nurses and advanced practice providers (APPs) to join us on our journey together to fight burnout and to find joy. Team Talk was included at the end of each chapter to apply the chapter's message to nurses and APPs. Lifting up physicians and all those who serve is the ultimate goal, and we cannot fail.

Journey Moments were added to stimulate thinking and to provide useful journaling exercises that will aid you on your climb to the summit. Think of them as base camp where great climbers rest, reflect, make decisions, and then decide to take positive strides forward in their upward ascent. Have a pen nearby, and try to complete each one.

"Self-help" was purposely included in the subtitle of the book, because it's the person you see in the mirror who ultimately holds the solutions and survival tactics to your own success. *Self*, when combined with commitment and hard work, is the prescription for burnout.

Begin the Journey

Now that you have opened *Fist Pumps: The Prescription for Physician Burnout*, before reading on I would like you to pause. Please take a moment to realize that choosing to read this book is the beginning of a journey that you have decided to take because you are determined to be joyful as a physician and healthcare provider. The book was written to inspire and motivate you to begin the amazing journey to your mountaintop of joy and fulfillment and equip you to say no to the valley of burnout. Whether inspired by a quote, a book, a song, or a YouTube video, don't underestimate the importance of making the decision to live and to practice differently.

I hope and pray that thousands of providers nationwide will regularly celebrate with a congratulatory fist pump as they live their journey loving and caring for our nation. Yes, please join the Fist Pumps Revolution and begin the journey to your mountaintop now! I hope you enjoy the book. Good luck to you all.

Part 1: The Crisis

CHAPTER 1

WE HAVE A HEALTHCARE CRISIS . . .
AND THE CRISIS IS NOW

I recently took a writing course at my local hospital. At week five's class, I raised my hand and asked the creative writing professor, "Why do people write?" What I was really trying to do was figure this out for myself. Why was I spending so much of my valuable time writing a book on healthcare when I had so many other things on my plate?

He looked me in the eye—and I will take his words to my grave—"Scott, people write because there's something they just have to say." For me it was a wow moment. It made so much sense. It was true.

Well, ladies and gentlemen, I wrote this book because there's something I just have to say: **We have a healthcare crisis . . . and the crisis is now.** Costs are soaring out of control, threatening the financial health of individuals and our nation. Quality of care is deteriorating, in spite of "world-class care" signs seemingly on every corner. And physicians are checking out and burning out. I believe it's one of the greatest societal issues of our day.

America currently spends more on healthcare than any other nation, estimated recently to be $3.6 trillion. According to the Centers for Medicare and Medicaid Services (CMS), we spend just over $11,000 annually per person on healthcare, up nearly 35 percent from twelve years previous. We more than double the per capita average spent by many other developed nations, and there's no end in sight.

But in the greatest country in the world who spends the most on healthcare, too many people cannot afford healthcare.

This includes not just the 30 million uninsured, but millions with insurance who have difficulty affording their deductibles and copays and are just one diagnosis away from financial peril. Monthly premiums are several hundred dollars and deductibles are anywhere from $2,000 to $10,000. And since the Affordable Care Act, people are experiencing annual rate hikes of 10 to 30 percent. In the face of declining paychecks and little family net worth, Americans cannot afford these staggering bills that, in many cases, are greater than their rent or home mortgages.

In the greatest country in the world who spends the most on healthcare, too many employers cannot afford healthcare as well.

Small businesses nationwide are struggling as their healthcare costs are rising. As a result, many are providing employees with less desirable coverage, raising employee contributions, and in many cases dropping coverage all together. Others are going out of business, not able to keep up with the expenses that are drowning them or surrendering to buyouts from larger businesses.

In the greatest country in the world who spends the most on healthcare, even the government cannot afford healthcare.

In spite of what your favorite politician or news channel might tell you, the government cannot afford Medicare and Medicaid. Simply put: government sponsored healthcare is going broke. If current spending continues, Medicare will be insolvent in a decade, according to the Medicare Trustees 2016 report. The national debt already exceeds $30 trillion. And healthcare spending, representing one-sixth of the nation's Gross Domestic Product, is a major driver of that debt. And it's only going to get worse with our aging and—let's face it, a tad on the chubby side—unhealthy population.

Show Me the Money

Let's pause for a moment and evaluate.

In the greatest country in the world who spends the most on healthcare, if the people don't have the money, and the employers don't have the money, and the government doesn't have the money, that leads me to asking, Jerry McGuire style, "Show me the money!" I really mean it: Who's got the money?

Over the years of building an absolutely fabulous healthcare system, we have over-corporatized the American healthcare system. The Wall Street players in medicine—those corporations that make the drugs and equipment, the hospitals, the legal profession, and the insurance industry—have got the money. And they're lobbying to the government daily to further fatten their war chests and maximize profits. They are doubling down year after year to ensure huge profit margins, driving the cost of healthcare further through the roof.

I'm not demonizing corporate America, and I don't want you to either. It's not bad to be successful, profitable, or answer to the stockholder. Corporate America has brought us one of the best healthcare systems in the world and I truly support their success. But unfortunately, when it comes to healthcare, it's gone too far.

It's Gone Too Far Because the Fallout Is Real

The fallout is real because the Main Street of medicine—the physician, the nurse, and the patient, or what I refer to as functional or day-to-day healthcare—is getting hammered. Physicians and nurses are overworked and stressed by the demands of the medical-industrial complex that demands they spend less time with patients who need them more. You can make a strong case now in America that the doctor, nurse, and patient exist so that a whole bunch of people can make a whole bunch of money off of them. One-sixth of the economy is printing cash from the healthcare industry, and we're paying for it—the patients and the providers. These high profits and costs associated are not sustainable.

And to make matters worse, Americans are not getting close to what they are paying for when it comes to healthcare. In spite of beautiful new hospitals with welcoming front lobbies and smiling greeters, many of the providers and workers in healthcare are less engaged, less knowledgeable, less empathetic, and too often don't do a very good job.

It's a complicated matter, but I believe that too much of our nursing care is not the quality it should be. Hospital administration has invested in expensive technology and treatments while cutting corners on the people actually working in medicine. Our healthcare system has invested in things, not people that care.

So what happens when you over-corporatize and commoditize healthcare, or perhaps better stated, you run healthcare like it's a big-box store? Guess what—you get a big-box store. It's highly functional, highly profitable, in many cases good or very good, but not excellent.

Corporatizing major industries is most often done to maximize profit through improved economy of scales, enhanced negotiating strength, and by monopolizing the landscape. Profit multiplies upward, but is rarely shared with the customer or end user. In fact, the end user often gets less. And in this case the end user is the patient, the physician, and other providers. Every day hospitals balance the fine line between delivering quality versus cutting costs to enhance profit, with a natural bias toward the latter.

And like our educational system, which I believe was commoditized decades ago, healthcare is now too ridiculously expensive, access by millions is limited, quality is deteriorating, the providers are devalued and disrespected, and in many cases, we're not getting what we pay for.

The Death Blow

Cost is a problem. Quality is a problem. **But the death blow to the American healthcare system will be the devaluation, the commoditization, and the gutting of the profession of medicine.** Because when the profession of medicine dies, the system dies.

And I say when physicians die the system dies, because we are the bridge to multi-million-dollar hospital profits. We are the bridge to using highly profitable drugs and equipment. We are the bridge to lowering insurance premiums by practicing cost-effective medicine. And most importantly, we are the bridge to providing loving, compassionate, and excellent healthcare.

Hear me out, America. Love is at the core of medical care. If we as physicians become commoditized and begin viewing ourselves as a profit center rather than a care provider, our great nation is going to be in a great deal of trouble.

The epidemic of physician burnout is a national crisis. The number of physicians checking out, wanting to leave the profession, or just make it to the finish line is unacceptable. As is the case with teachers, a nation suffers when those representing such an important pillar of society burn out and lose their purpose of helping others and serving. And for what gain will we allow this to happen, greed and money?

My love for this country and for my profession will not allow this to happen without sounding the alarm.

So, ladies and gentlemen. I wrote this book because *we have a healthcare crisis . . . and the crisis is now.*

TEAM TALK

Nurses and advanced practice providers are well aware of our healthcare crisis. Manning the front lines and caring for our nation, they are similarly overworked, stressed, and burning out in record numbers.

COVID-19 has thrown fuel on the burnout fire, but the crisis has existed for years. Nurses and advanced practice providers are wanting to leave their profession, retiring, or job-hopping for extra dollars. Morale is at a low point and the quality of care has been affected by the nursing shortage.

I love the profession of nursing and deeply respect advanced practice providers. The country has been blessed by having so many amazing providers. By sounding the alarm and writing this book, I hope that some of these words will be uplifting and beneficial to them.

A JOURNEY MOMENT

Do you believe that we have a healthcare crisis?

_____

_____

_____

_____

_____

_____

Do you think that healthcare has been over-corporatized?

_____

_____

_____

_____

_____

_____

Has your joy in practicing medicine been negatively impacted as a result?

_____
_____
_____
_____
_____
_____

Is physician and provider burnout a concern or interest of yours?

_____
_____
_____
_____
_____
_____

Do you long to be inspired and excited by being a healthcare provider?

_____
_____
_____
_____
_____
_____

If you said yes to a number of these questions, please read on.
We have a journey to take—together.

CHAPTER 2

SITTING POOLSIDE . . . WHAT I BELIEVE

It was my daughter Lindsey's spring break, and the family just wanted to get away, get a tan, and do nothing. After back-to-back years of wearing jackets to shield us from the cool, crisp winds on Isle of Palms during spring break, we were desperate for heat. Charleston is one of the nicest destinations on the planet, but unfortunately, its weather can be a little bit nippy in early April. We were ready for muscles on muscles, some New Jersey trash talk, blistered feet on scorching walkways, and my favorite summer beverage: orange-pineapple with dark rum and a lot of ice. Fort Lauderdale Hilton poolside—here we come!

It was seven days of blue skies, Jimmy Buffett, delicious seafood, and a full packet of antacids. The Florida strip was no disappointment. But the sixth-floor infinity pool was jam-packed, and for us to get poolside, Lindsey and I had to get up early to claim our territory. With towels creased into lounge-chair backs, flip flops and beach bags laid across, and my computer case nearby, we regularly found a spot that provided us an excellent vantage point of sun, ocean, and sights.

With a cherry-red shoulder and a burnt forehead victimized by my fresh military-style buzz cut and an aversion to hats, on day two I was already getting antsy. To the observant, one can always pick out the type As, the workaholics, and yes, the folks that just can't truly relax unless they are "doing something," even on their well-needed and longed-for vacation. Guilty as charged, with a gentle sigh and concealed smile, I cracked opened my computer.

I started writing down a number of ideas that eventually became this book, etching in stone my beliefs about healthcare. Beliefs that have never changed and I predict never will.

I think it's important for readers to know these beliefs, since our beliefs are the prism through which we see and interpret the world. They shape our thoughts and words, and mine may be very different from yours.

When it comes to healthcare, I believe:

1. A great nation is a healthy nation.
2. In a great nation, every living soul should go to bed at night feeling safe knowing they have access to excellent and affordable healthcare.
3. In a great nation, excellence is more important than profit, especially when it comes to healthcare.
4. In a great nation, the best and brightest young men and women should yearn, and I mean yearn, to be healthcare providers, as I did growing up in eastern Canada.
5. And, I believe that in a great nation, physicians and those called to serve are different, and the health and well-being of the nation rests on their shoulders.

Writing makes you think. It makes you dig deep and go places that our busy world and hectic schedules won't normally allow. It forces you to question your soul about what really matters. Writing makes you ask yourself what words you are hoping to engrave in history, and who you are trying to impact.

I came to realize what truly drives me. I came to realize my vision, my lofty goal. A lofty goal is one that you'll pursue forever, knowing it can never be reached or fully satisfied. A goal that hopefully inspires others to pursue as well, with the hope that we can increase our impact together, but more importantly—impact future generations.

Simply stated, my lofty goal is to create a world that lifts up physicians and other healthcare providers who serve. *A world that nourishes and brings joy* *and fulfillment to those who serve and help others. The health and well-being of our nation depends on it.*

I've realized that I must speak up and reach out to like-minded physicians, nurses, APPs, and other providers. Unified, we can help and support one another, we can encourage, and we can rescue the greatest profession ever bestowed upon humans: the profession of medicine.

Perhaps you've listened to Martin Luther King's "I Have a Dream" speech. If not, I highly recommend it. Back then, the civil rights movement did not have social media, the internet, or an advertising budget, and yet 250,000 civil rights supporters sharing a similar dream travelled great distances and participated in that historic day on August 28, 1963, in Washington DC. Thousands of like-minded people with a similar dream were all present to help and support one another and foster encouragement. All present became a unified voice to make a positive impact.

My dream is a world that lifts up healthcare providers and encourages them to live out their calling, to live out their why. To use their gifts and talents to help others. A world where burnout is non-existent. Helping the person to your right, and then to the left, is the perfect and divine plan for all.

I dream of a world where everyone who serves is proud of themselves, and they will fight for the stamina and discipline necessary to bear such tremendous responsibility. It is this same responsibility that when realized, empowers them to be successful in their journey. To be successful in reaching their mountaintop, that sacred place where you find joy, peace, virtue, and contentment. It's where life gives you meaning and purpose.

I dream of a world in which millions of like-minded people will come together and experience their August 28, 1963, moment. They will come together to help and support each other, and with a unified voice make a positive impact regarding healthcare, physician joy, and burnout. We need inspiration. We need hope. We need each other.

I encourage those who serve to look up to God or a higher power, or to look inward for strength, but to realize that you are different: you've been asked to serve. You've been asked to sacrifice. You've been asked to reach beyond yourself for others. And I believe only the best respond to that calling, and only the best are given that privilege.

It's poolside, day seven. Unfortunately, the moments enjoying the blue skies, Jimmy Buffett, and the sixth-floor infinity pool have come to an end for us. It's time to go back to work for me, and back to school for Lindsey.

We've all got work to do. We've all got dreams to live and fulfill. So let's get started—together.

Team Talk

The health and well-being of the nation rests on the shoulders of healthcare providers, including nurses and advanced practice providers. They too have been called to use their gifts and talents to help others.

We need all providers to be joyful and fulfilled when caring for patients. Their mission to serve is vital, and they need to be lifted up and supported. The pressure placed on nurses and APPs as a result of over-commoditizing healthcare is intense and mounting.

But together, we can help and encourage one another to live out our purpose, to live out our why. Together, we can have our August 28, 1963, moment.

A Journey Moment

How are your beliefs concerning healthcare similar to or different from mine?

_____

_____

_____

_____

Would the country benefit from lifting up physicians and other healthcare providers?

_____

_____

_____

_____

_____

_____

Do you have a lofty goal in either your personal or professional life?

_____

_____

_____

_____

_____

Now, or while reading this book, write down your lofty goal or goals. Maybe you know it right away, or maybe you just have an inkling and need time to think about it, or maybe they fall somewhere in-between, but write them down. It's a beneficial exercise.

My lofty goal(s) is/are:

_____

_____

_____

_____

_____

_____

_____

_____

CHAPTER 3

BURNOUT INVENTORY

Are you a "noticer?" Andy Andrews is a hilarious motivational speaker and author of *The Traveler's Gift*, and believes that a small percentage of the population are noticers. They can spot things that others don't.

They notice that rusty window frame resulting from sloppy construction. Those overgrown shrubs in front of a struggling business. They notice the employee's smile, quietly announcing that she's in love and that she may want to share her feelings with others but is too embarrassed.

As a card-carrying noticer, I can vouch that it's advantageous to be aware of one's surroundings, but at times it can feel like a curse. Just going with the flow might be a welcome reprieve from the moments of frustration that a noticer must endure.

For years, I've noticed a change in my fellow physicians. Gradual, insidious, but yes, a definite change.

Those once strong and confident, many at the top of their game, no longer walk around with their chests out proudly, but walk with their shoulders slumped. Caring smiles have been replaced by faces prematurely aged by stress. I've noticed short tempers, fewer caring words, and less laughter. I've noticed the best are palpably frustrated, bitter, and resentful; many have checked out emotionally, or are just trying to get to retirement. Just recently, two friends of mine retired early, saying that they were no longer willing to put up with the endless frustrations of practicing medicine and that their happiness was too important. Perhaps reacting to declining reimbursement or other stressors, but I've noticed that too many physicians commoditize their patients in an attempt to enrich themselves.

We have a word for these changes: burnout.

The History of Burnout

Early in her career, Christina Maslach, a clinical social psychologist from the University of California, Berkeley, was fascinated by her research interviewing people in the workplace and exploring what emotional challenges they might be experiencing.

In particular, she noted that those working in human services, healthcare, and education are often required to spend considerable time in intense interactions with others. These people are often burdened and share a number of psychological, social, or physical problems. She consistently found that those who worked with people under these circumstances experienced chronic stress that was emotionally draining and led to burnout.

Maslach, coauthor of the "Maslach Burnout Inventory," described burnout as an "erosion of the soul caused by a deterioration of one's values, dignity, spirit, and will." It's a psychological syndrome comprised of emotional exhaustion, depersonalization, and reduced personal accomplishment.

Emotional exhaustion is when you're so physically and emotionally wiped, you don't know if you can go back to work. You don't know how much longer you can continue. Your physical and emotional energy is depleted, especially the energy needed to share and interact with others.

Most days I find myself energized, but I pause to think of my colleagues who feel physically or emotionally exhausted. I remember how drained I feel after finishing a really bad weekend on call, and wonder if that is how they must feel, but all the time. Man, that would be rough, especially in a job like medicine that demands so much energy and attentiveness.

When you depersonalize your job, you become overly cynical, sarcastic, and get up on your soapbox when talking about your patients, job, and career. I'm the soapboxer in chief, or at least I once was. It's when the patient becomes more like a number and a means to an end rather than a person with whom you would like to solve their physical ailments. Emotionally tapped, you're no longer available for a healthy connection.

When you stop believing in what you do, you decrease your sense of personal accomplishment. You stop believing in your why. You no longer see your purpose as a healthcare provider. After giving my life to my career, I can't imagine feeling that way, but many do and dream of an escape from their daily realities.

Loss of Joy

There have been a number of different terms applied to physician burnout. Recently, experts have referred to it as "moral injury," and in many ways I agree with that terminology. Moral injury, or post-traumatic stress, was first used to describe soldiers' responses to actions in war. These soldiers bore witness to acts and situations that violated their moral beliefs and expectations.

In medicine, many providers experience similar injury when they feel that they're no longer able to adequately care for their patients as a result of their environment. Pulled in so many directions by the business of medicine, many stop believing in the process. Importantly, this demoralization is a result of a broken healthcare system, not due to an individual's inability to cope or their lack of resilience.

But no matter its name—burnout, or moral injury, or other—the fundamental problem is a loss of joy. I've always considered medicine as a profession of joy, perhaps like no other. Medicine is the perfect mosaic combining one's calling, sacrifice, challenges, skills, and using one's gifts to help others. It's truly a transcendent design.

I believe that healthcare providers in the past were blessed with full joy tanks. The first several years of my practice were wonderful. Patients were trusting and appreciative. The quality of the nursing care was excellent. There was less financial pressure, allowing me to spend more time with patients. But especially in the last decade, the system keeps taking from us, and taking from us, and taking from us. And we just keep refilling the tank, and refilling the tank, and at some point we can no longer keep refilling the tank. And now the joy meter for many is running low, and for others their joy tank is empty. This loss of joy is a serious problem for our profession, for healthcare, and for our nation.

The Burnout Fact Sheet

In the general population, the incidence of occupational burnout is 28 percent. In physicians, it's almost twofold higher: 54 percent. And the trend, unfortunately, may be rising, and the COVID-19 pandemic has only made it worse. In a 2020 Medscape survey, 64 percent of physicians said that the pandemic had intensified their sense of burnout.

Burnout rates across specialties show only minor differences, and the prevalence in primary care, resident physicians, and those employed versus those in private practice is similar. Midcareer providers may be the most susceptible, and the data evaluating gender differences varies.

Many physicians suffer in silence. They are embarrassed, they are afraid of being belittled by partners or ignored by the large healthcare system that employs them. They fear mental health disclosures could jeopardize their licenses or adversely affect their disability insurance. Many are living in a valley of anger, bitterness, resentment, and a multitude of other negative emotions that we'll discuss.

In a study of full-time academic physicians and scientists, one in five reported significant depressive symptoms, with higher levels in younger faculty. In a survey of almost 8,000 practicing surgeons, 38 percent had symptoms of depression, and 6 percent reported thoughts of suicide in the year prior.

Compared with other professions, physicians' proportionate mortality ratio from suicide is 1.5 to 4.5 times higher than the rest of the population. Three to four hundred physicians commit suicide annually. That's unacceptable—it's the equivalent to a Boeing 747 going down every year full of doctors who are suffering.

Excellence in healthcare not only relies on physicians, but on a team of highly dedicated and compassionate providers. Forty to forty-nine percent of registered nurses experience burnout as well, and nearly one-half of newly-licensed nurses leave their first job within three years. It appears that the high burnout rate amongst APPs is similar to other primary care providers.

Why Should I Care?

I think that many outside the medical profession may be surprised or even empathetic upon learning about physician burnout, but they might have other thoughts, like "me too." Thoughts of "join the crowd," or "they should hear my story," and "why should I care?"

Let's face it, it's common to have workplace problems. So many of our major industries have over-corporatized, and workers have been purposely devalued and overworked. Devaluation promotes a culture where workers are paid less, are required to be more obedient, and they become a replaceable cog on the wheel of corporate America. Racing humans to the bottom in an attempt to increase profits is a well-established business strategy. In addition, regardless of workplace circumstances, everyone is burdened by the same personal, family, and societal stresses. Unfortunately, burnout has become endemic.

But we should be cautious when thinking about physician and healthcare provider burnout, because there's a critical difference. When people who serve others in their profession are devalued, commoditized, and check out, it's not good for society, and it's not good for you. The health of a great nation rests on the shoulders of those who serve—our teachers, police officers, firefighters, military, healthcare providers, and more.

I have seen this before with the profession of teaching. During my fellowship at Duke, I often reflected about education in America, as it differed so much from the Canadian system. I wondered why, in the greatest and richest country in the world (and trust me America was really wealthy in the early nineties and relatively debt free), did society allow one of its most important generational assets—the teaching system—to die?

Did anyone care that many kids were not getting a good education or the proper resources to succeed? Did the country really think that the best and the brightest would sign up for a career of teaching, which would pay them mediocre salaries, and in return, families and students could devalue them and be disrespectful to them? Did the private school crowd's "it's not my problem" philosophy somehow shelter the country from the perils of having a less educated, less informed, and now a less disciplined, entitled society?

Did this destruction to such a precious commodity happen overnight, or was it a slow, insidious process?

Burnout in physicians negatively impacts quality of care and significantly contributes to medical errors. Dissatisfied providers are less productive and more likely to leave their practice or choose early retirement. Turnover is costly. Apathy multiplies and excellence declines. The occurrence of medical errors and associated increased patient dissatisfaction are known predictors of malpractice litigation.

The end result is that quality deteriorates. Costs and premiums skyrocket. The cogs multiply. With the trajectory of each, unfortunately, all are heading in the wrong direction. And sadly, there are not enough noticers to speak up and to sound the alarm.

Psychologist and researcher Christina Maslach is right: burnout is an erosion of the soul caused by a deterioration of one's values, dignity, spirit, and will. It's an enormous problem for physicians. It's an enormous problem for healthcare and for our country.

Burnout, moral injury, loss of joy. Regardless of its nomenclature, it's a really big deal. But only you can decide what you think. And only you can decide if you care.

TEAM TALK

Statistics shining the light on nurse burnout are everywhere.

- 98 percent of hospital nurses reported their work to be mentally and physically demanding, and 63 percent suffered from burnout.
- About one-third of nurses surveyed reported an emotional exhaustion score that qualified them as "high burnout."
- 43.4 percent of nurses are considering leaving their current jobs, citing burnout as an underlying cause.
- Approximately 40 percent of critical care nurses nationwide reported depressive symptoms, and 50 percent experienced anxiety. These poor health scores directly correlated with an increase in self-reported medical errors.
- Almost half a million registered nurses had already left their profession nationwide, citing high workloads, limited staffing, and forced to work "voluntary overtime" as reasons for departure.
- 62 percent of nurses report that the national nursing shortage is already strongly impacting them.
- The incidence of nurse burnout has dramatically escalated as a result of COVID-19.

Similar data exists for advanced practice providers:

- The average burnout rate for APPs in the United States is 32.6 percent.
- Burnout symptoms are key contributors to both depression and medical errors among APPs.
- 46 percent of APPs studied met the criteria for work exhaustion and 30 percent for interpersonal disengagement.
- 40 percent of APPs showed symptoms of burnout and the COVID-19 pandemic has increased rates of anxiety.

Reading these burnout fact sheets should bring us pause. It saddens me that my colleagues on the front lines are being so adversely affected. Physicians have witnessed the physical and emotional wear and tear on our nurses and advanced practice providers resulting from COVID-19.

Nurse and APP burnout is a really big deal. And we all need to care.

A JOURNEY MOMENT

Have you noticed a change in physician demeanor, words, and/or behavior in the last number of years? If yes, how?

_____

_____

_____

_____

_____

_____

_____

_____

_____

Looking in the mirror, have you noticed a change in you that might be a symptom of burnout? If yes, list up to five of those changes.

1. _____

2. _____

3. _____

4. _____

5. _____

Chapter 4

The Causes of Burnout

Being a healthcare provider, I suppose it's not surprising that I'm often asked why physicians burn out. My initial response is always the same: "You're kidding me, right?"

Well, let me explain. First, it's important to understand the makeup of most physicians. Their left brain is the side of perfectionism, of "the buck stops with me," of "just get the job done," and excellence. When you combine those qualities with their right brain of love, compassion, and caring—that's their love language. Then take that human being whose profession was once one that garnered respect, gratitude, and trust for a job well done, and you put that person into today's healthcare system? That's like leading a lamb to the slaughter.

Today's healthcare system is like a death by a thousand cuts for physicians. Whether it's electronic medical records, the next pre-authorization, another rule or regulation, the list goes on. And day after day, year after year, those cuts can really wear you down.

Just as restaurant owners struggle to give a good dining experience to their customers with inadequate staffing, we are trying to provide excellent care to patients with a fragmented team that in many cases is not capable of delivering excellence. Not even close, and it's incredibly frustrating.

Hospital administrators have sacrificed us for profit. And too often, we don't believe in what they believe, and we don't necessarily trust or respect them.

There's no loyalty, no trust. That's a very difficult environment. It's no wonder burnout is a problem.

We work in a healthcare system that has seriously hurt doctors financially. Some of the smartest and hardest working men and women—highly educated, taking on such tremendous responsibilities, multitasking through lunch, working long hours—are having difficulty affording their own private practices. And as a result, many have forfeited their practice and control over to more expensive hospital systems, increasing the cost to all. Unbelievable; shame on the endless Medicare cuts in reimbursement for allowing this to happen.

I don't think many speak to this, and perhaps I'm not politically correct enough, but the patients are killing us too. The loss of civility of our nation in the last two decades truly saddens and discourages me. We experience rudeness, anger, and endless demands in my waiting room and in interactions with my staff and myself daily. There's no place for it in medicine. Belittling front-desk staff, refusing to pay their bills, yelling at nurses over the phone, demands for their prescriptions to be called in, and blaming physicians that they are not getting better begins every Monday morning when the doors open.

The patient-physician relationship—the relationship of trust, respect, and feeling valued—has been commoditized into "How much does it cost?" and patient happiness or satisfaction is based on its outcome. When the relationship is destroyed like this, you just took a knife and thrust it into my love language, the right side of my brain.

This behavior attacks the fundamental reason why I practice medicine: to have a mutually respectful relationship where I can offer my help and try to do my best. You're attacking my why. If this is only going to be a left-brain relationship, the practice of medicine may not be for me. I might as well work on Wall Street and trade stocks and bonds.

For the most part, these things in healthcare are happening out of the control of doctors, and that loss of control is the kiss of death in compounding the problem and promoting burnout. Yes, that loss of control is helping lead that lamb to the slaughter.

The cause of burnout is multifactorial, with many factors affecting individuals differently. Let's address some more causes.

Work First, Life Second

The seeds of physician burnout are planted early during our training. Long hours, endless workloads, and a lack of control over schedules indoctrinate us with habits that are counterproductive to achieving critical life balance.

In residency, many cope by putting their personal lives on hold under the guise of "delayed gratification." But many maintain this habit in their practice as well, and rather than reclaiming their personal lives, they delay starting a family, nourishing hobbies outside of work, and time spent with family even longer, and in many cases indefinitely. Work comes first, life second. This is an existence sadly seen as normal.

A Lost Profession

Many physicians feel that we've lost the profession of medicine. The profession of knowledge, autonomy, nobility, and ethical constraints. We have a profession, not a job. We have patients, not customers. We have relationships, we don't have business transactions.

Our profession is sacred. Its sanctity is so much greater than individual physicians, no matter their accomplishments. A sanctity that has benefitted and inspired societies for generations.

It's discouraging that we are losing the profession of medicine and that it has been so devalued and disrespected by corporatized healthcare. It's demoralizing that it's been commoditized. It's sad and frustrating to be just a cog in the wheel of the medical industrial complex. It took me a long time to realize that this was the primary source of my bitterness and resentment.

To be devalued by third-party payers, the government, and litigation attorneys is arguably not worth fussing about because we are physically and emotionally distant from them. But when hospitals sacrifice physicians and providers in attempts to satisfy patients and meet reimbursable metrics, that's a tough pill to swallow. When patients are the valued customer, no matter how impossible, how demanding, how mean-spirited to providers, and the physicians and nurses come last, there's something wrong with the system.

Historically, physicians worked hand in hand with administrators and were the functional voice of most hospitals. Now they're a means to an end, worker bees, and quite frankly, a thorn in the side of many administrators. If you don't believe me, just ask their consultants. The consultants that administrators hire to help streamline their hospitals wouldn't give a second thought to a lost profession because they view medicine as a commodity from which to make money and don't value those who are delivering the care.

Financial Stress

Many physicians are under too much financial stress. They receive lower reimbursement from third-party payers, and yet their overhead continues to increase. As a result, there are more faded carpets, outdated computers, and aging clinics visibly apparent to all. Staff salaries are stagnant and quarterly bonuses have become a distant memory. Let's face it, the good old days of financial prosperity for many doctors are over.

The financial stress is to some degree a result of their own doing. Some physicians might have expectations of a larger paycheck that used to be true in past years, and their lifestyle has not been adjusted to match current realities. And as we'll discuss under solutions and survival tactics, slowing down and trading money for having margin in your work schedule and less stress is a very important strategy in battling burnout. But without attitudinal and lifestyle adjustments, the math may not add up.

The Pressure is Palpable

Burnout expert Dike Drummond, MD, author of *Stop Physician Burnout,* regularly states that the practice of medicine is stressful. "We are dealing with hurt, sick, scared, dying people, and their families." That's a lot of emotional burden to bear, especially on a regular basis.

But overall, it's a smaller contributor than other factors. I believe that most of us are very capable of handling such stress, and many actually thrive on this responsibility. But over time, this emotional burden could erode even the strongest of souls.

What I think has compounded this stress exponentially—well beyond the patient's diagnosis, treatment, and prognosis—is the patient's expectations and their loss of civility, as noted.

As a reconstructive surgeon who treats bladder and pelvic floor dysfunction, many of my patients who don't reach their treatment goals with surgery can be quite upset and don't mind letting you know. There's anger when surgery fails. If the patient experiences a complication, there's finger-pointing and telling others that you messed them up. Taking personal responsibility that they consented to a procedure knowing that it might not help them and understanding it has risks is not in their vocabulary. And if not them, their family members don't mind being the messenger. All of this behavior is independent of age, socio-economic status, and occurs even after a thorough preoperative consent and counseling that sets expectations about potential outcomes.

We live in an outcome-based commoditized society engineered by others to drive consumerism and profit, and medicine is no exception. The pressure we're under for "perfect" outcomes, especially as surgeons, is palpable. Only in this country does a surgeon regularly cross his fingers on opening a letter from an attorney or when entering the room to visit with a complicated postoperative patient. Unlike coaches, when it comes to surgery, the losing physician does not get a second season. Complications and poor outcomes have now become unacceptable; someone is always to blame.

EMR

One can't mention physician burnout without talking about electronic medical records (EMR). Unlike many industries in which technology improves efficiency, EMR has increased our clerical burden and distracts us from meaningful interactions with patients. Advertised as a means of eliminating transcription costs, EMR forced doctors to become data entry personnel.

But less commonly spoken of is its unacceptable performance and functionality. Certainly until recently, EMR would never compete or be acceptable to other industries or the public. I sometimes speculate that planes would be falling out of the sky if the airline industry relied upon similar technology. In my experience, "going live" with the next EMR update is always a source of frustration and stress.

EMR software programs and infrastructure seemed to be introduced into the complex world of healthcare much too early. Healthcare functioned as a living beta site for decades. And now the system is paying billions for fixing the mess that should never have been implemented in the first place. Almost daily, the EMR program in our clinic malfunctions or doesn't interface well with the hospital system. And to make matters worse for physicians, the cost associated with implementation, maintenance, and upgrades, and the loss of productivity associated is staggering. Our practice of fifteen providers pays approximately $300,000 annually for IT support and electronic medical records.

EMR is an enormous business influenced and regulated by industry, government, consultants, and lobbyists. A business forced upon physicians, nurses, and healthcare nationwide. Wall Street wins. Main Street loses. There's no question that EMR has increased physician burnout.

On Call

Perhaps one of the greatest stressors to many physicians is being on call. In fact, it's a common reason why many surgeons retire early. Answering pages and working twenty-four hours straight or longer is tiresome and stressful. Only surgeons can appreciate the burden of operating on sick patients in the middle of the night and returning to work the next morning.

While physicians know that this is part of the job description when they go into medicine, things have changed about how often we're contacted. Years ago, specialists were rarely paged during the night. But with commoditized health-care and emergency departments now busy 24-7, they're regularly called around the clock. Emergency room physicians and nurse practitioners, hospital floor nurses, all who can go home at the end of their shifts, call specialists endlessly with little regard to their health or sleep. Just last night I was called at three in the morning by the ER—only to tell me they were sending a patient home with instructions to call our office for follow-up. I did not need to be notified of that. Soon after, a hospital nurse paged me for an order of a medication that clearly could have waited until morning. Many of the calls are not necessary. Many of the calls and consults could wait. And many of the calls would never happen in other countries.

The nighttime wear and tear of being on call is taking its toll on many.

Breaking Point

It's easy to blame others for physician burnout, but we need to take stock of our own culpability, which we'll discuss in chapter 13 when we "rethink the battle." Like most complicated issues, there's more than one side to the story.

The stresses of medicine don't occur in isolation. I don't know about you, but I find life in general pretty stressful. Social media, the news, our phones, the pace, all of us trying to do more with less time—it's all very taxing.

In addition, most people are or will experience a significant personal, family, or close-friend crisis, whether it's emotional, physical, financial, or other. In an ideal world, our personal life is the place where we get recharged, but in many cases, we go home to additional sources of stress.

There's no question that the cause of burnout and loss of joy in our profession is multi-factorial. Those stressors continue to add up and pile

on, so that even one of the most resilient populations—physicians—have reached their breaking point.

TEAM TALK

Nurses and advanced practice providers identify with the many causes of burnout: death by a thousand cuts, trying to deliver excellent care while working with a fragmented team, being sacrificed for profit, increasing financial stress, and caring for difficult patients is experienced by many.

Other sources include long hours, ever-increasing workloads, limited staffing, forced overtime, too many nonclinical duties, difficult colleagues, and feeling underappreciated.

Without a voice or control, providers feel demoralized, especially when the patient—the "customer"—comes first. With multiple burnout factors being endlessly piled on, many nurses and APPs have finally reached their breaking point and are moving on to greener pastures.

A JOURNEY MOMENT

Can you identify with any of the causes of physician burnout? If yes, list your top five:

1. _____
2. _____
3. _____
4. _____
5. _____

Do you feel that some of the causes are beginning to pile on and are adversely affecting your joy and fulfillment as a healthcare provider? If so, when is it time to do something about it? (Please read on . . .)

_____

_____

Chapter 5

The Descent into the Valley of Burnout

Burnout is like living in a valley. And it's important for each of us to have a deep appreciation of what that valley looks like. **Because the realization that you don't want to live there, and that your family and others around you don't want you to live there, is an important, actionable step in fighting and preventing burnout.**

There appears to be stages of burnout that gradually worsen the further down into the valley. The deeper you go, the more adversely you're affected, as are others around you.

Early into the descent are feelings of frustration, irritation, and as I sometimes jokingly say, being "chronically annoyed." Death by a thousand cuts, struggling with a fragmented team, unhappy patients: I think one could make a strong case for who wouldn't be annoyed.

When we're annoyed and frustrated, we complain, we criticize, we get up on our soapboxes, and from time to time, we lose our cool. But for the most part, if we can rest and recover over the weekend, we rebound, have minimal long-term sequelae, and are still reasonably content and fulfilled. Perhaps some of you fit this description.

It was at this point in the valley where I lived for a number of years. But looking back, I now realize my tolerance to such annoyances, such mediocrity, such disrespect and devaluation lessened over time. And it was to my detriment. Looking back, I didn't nip it in the bud and deal with the issues. Insidiously, I descended further into the valley, losing more of the good in me and acquiring more of the bad.

Deeper in the valley, many physicians find themselves living in a world of bitterness, anger, and what I ultimately had to face: resentment. Yes, resentment lives within our profession and it's not good, not good for anyone.

Resentment can be destructive. Short-tempered, easily angered, barking and biting, cynical cutting sarcasm doled out to employees and administrators. For some, it's about commoditizing patients, listening less, caring less, trading excellence for apathy. And sadly, sometimes the overprescribing of financially rewarding tests, procedures, and surgery.

I now realize that the ill effects of bitterness and resentment do not live in isolation, nor do they live only within the walls of my work. The same bark, the same short temperament and criticism adversely affected my relationship at home with my wife Andrea and my daughter Lindsey.

A few years ago, I was bitter and resentful because it was unacceptable to me that the profession of medicine was so devalued and disrespected, even by patients. My negative thinking, superimposed on the other stressors that healthcare providers endure, really made me angry. I allowed my thoughts to change me from being a pretty happy and positive person, to one who was negative, sarcastic, and judgmental.

Initially my family provided me grace and encouragement, since they understood the stress and burden that I was dealing with. But my chronic negativity finally wore them down. Andrea and Lindsey spoke to me about my behavior, and I decided that night that I was going to change. No longer was I going to sacrifice my relationship with family for my career. I guess you could say that I had my Andrea and Lindsey moment. The people who loved me the most saved me from myself. Yes, it was my turning point.

Hear me loud and clear: when you're burned out and joy and fulfillment are absent, it affects so many—your family, your friends, your patients, and

many others around you. Everyone suffers. Yes, everyone is pulled down into the valley. Don't wait for your Andrea and Lindsey moment. Say no to the valley of burnout now.

The deepest descent into the valley of burnout is the path that takes you to a place of discouragement, fearfulness, loneliness, and loss of hope. These are places that, fortunately, I've never ventured. You stop believing in your purpose. You stop believing in your why and what you've given your life for. Some are so deeply tortured they may call it hell. And as we've learned, too many resort to suicide.

TEAM TALK

The descent into the valley of burnout is experienced by nurses and advanced practice providers. Early in the descent, they regularly feel frustrated, fatigued, and stressed by the dysfunctional healthcare system. Many hope just to get through the day without experiencing too much strain and suffering. They refuel on days off only to return to the same environment.

Deeper in the valley, many nurses and APPs are angry and resentful. They are short-tempered, sarcastic, and openly criticize their employer and teammates. Gossip and finger-pointing is common and destructive to all. Bitterness doesn't have an on/off switch, and relationships at home suffer.

Apathy multiplies and checked-out providers begin accepting their own mediocrity. Excellence and "the buck stops with me" is replaced by "no one else cares, so why should I?" Quality deteriorates and patient care suffers as the system self-destructs. And job-hopping for a few extra dollars becomes a new norm.

Deepest in the valley of burnout, many feel lonely and discouraged. They are exhausted by the endless shifts without having enough staff. Watching another COVID-19 patient die from respiratory failure with no family present is a cross that many can no longer bear.

Cries for help to administration go unnoticed, but many providers dread telling their spouses that they are miserable and just want to quit. "How will I look after my family and what is my plan B?" are the words of the fearful and desperate.

Nationwide, nurses and advanced practice providers are anxious and depressed as they struggle with their calling to use their gifts to help others. No longer believing in their purpose is confusing and can torture even the strongest. And as is the case with physicians, too many nurses and APPs succumb to hopelessness and even suicide.

A JOURNEY MOMENT

Do you believe that there are stages to burnout?

_____

_____

_____

_____

_____

Do you think burnout happens quickly, or is it slow and insidious?

_____

_____

_____

_____

Have you descended into the valley of burnout?

_____

_____

_____

_____

_____

If yes, where in the valley do you currently find yourself?

_____

_____

_____

_____

_____

Does your burnout need to be addressed? Are there issues or concerns that need to be nipped in the bud?

_____

_____

_____

_____

_____

A CHALLENGE

Regarding yourself, ask a friend or loved one the last three questions. Please listen to their answers. Their words may be life-changing to you and to those around you. Taking this brave step may be just what's necessary to initiate your journey.

CHAPTER 6

"HOUSTON, WE HAVE A PROBLEM"

John Swigert, Jr., James Lovell, and Fred Haise, Jr.—the crew of the Apollo 13 moon flight on April 14, 1970—reported a problem back to NASA Mission Control. "Okay, Houston, we've had a problem here." The spacecraft was malfunctioning, caused by an explosion and rupture of an oxygen tank in the service module. The subsequent loss of oxygen resulted in the crew having to abort the mission.

The survival of the crew was on everyone's conscience. With all hands on deck, NASA was determined to rescue the three and bring them home safely. And against all odds, they did.

"Houston, we have a problem" is a common but erroneous quotation popularized by the 1995 film, a dramatization of the Apollo 13 mission. To this day, this phrase is regularly used to indicate a major problem.

Well ladies and gentlemen, when it comes to healthcare, "Houston, we have a problem." Costs are soaring, quality is deteriorating, physicians are both burning out and checking out. It is one of the most important societal issues of our day.

And as was the case with Apollo that was coined the "86 hours of terror" and the greatest space rescue in history engineered by the masterful minds of NASA, we, too, must work together on a common mission to save our healthcare system and rescue the physicians and those who serve.

Now that we've looked at the issues, we'll discuss solutions and survival tactics to not only fight burnout, but more importantly, to find joy and fulfillment as a healthcare provider. I remember the pain I felt in telling my wife Andrea that I wanted to go to work feeling fulfilled and inspired and not so burned out.

In our journey together we'll talk about climbing out of the valley and ascending to our mountaintop, and the meaning life provides when standing on the summit. We'll visit with the desperate lows in the valley of burnout and make conscious decisions that the valley is not where we want to live.

We'll learn that fulfillment is actually experienced just by looking up out of the valley and choosing to make the difficult ascent to the summit. **Yes, even just the decision and attempt to climb often brings more fulfillment in the midst of a problem than not having the problem to begin with.** Don't underestimate the power of looking up. There is power in determination and power in pride.

In discussing solutions and survival tactics, I will call on each of us to *be different.* In doing so, we can make mountaintop decisions and ascend the steep path to the summit and battle the epidemic of physician burnout so common in the valley. And by being different, I believe we physicians can make a positive impact in fixing our healthcare crisis.

As you visualize your climb to the summit, the journey may appear daunting. It may look too steep, too difficult, too overwhelming to those who are in the valley just trying to survive. But ahead lies dreams of joy, contentment, significance as a spouse, as a parent or friend, as a physician. For some, "Can I ever experience these dreams again?" may be a fair question.

Well, I believe, as was the case with Apollo 13, that against tremendous odds, the answer is yes. Haise, Lovell, and Swigert splashed down safely at 12:07 p.m. on April 17, 1970, and so you, too, can be pulled from your command module onto a life-saving raft. You too can look up, be proud, and finish strong.

TEAM TALK

"Houston, we have a problem," can easily be applied to nurses and APPs. Costs are soaring, quality is deteriorating, and many nurses and advanced practice providers are burning out and checking out, threatening the health of our nation. They are an integral part of our healthcare system, and they must be happy and healthy in order to serve.

In our journey together we will discuss solutions and survival tactics to fight burnout and to be joyful and fulfilled. We will encourage and support one another and ascend to our mountaintop and finish strong.

A JOURNEY MOMENT

If you are experiencing burnout, does your climb to the summit appear daunting?

_____

_____

_____

If yes, why? (I encourage you to give this question a lot of thought. Identifying circumstances, barriers, and personal struggles that are weighing you down is a critical step in becoming a good climber.)

_____

_____

_____

_____

_____

_____

_____

_____

_____

_____

Part 2: Successful Battle Strategies in the Fight Against Burnout

Chapter 7

The Battle Against Burnout

When I was first invited to speak to my colleagues on healthcare, I primarily addressed the decline of our healthcare system as a result of its over-corporatization and the gutting of the profession of medicine.

As a result of these talks, I was often requested to speak more about the physician burnout side of the story. Listeners identified with and agreed with the healthcare crisis, but they were looking for solutions to their own daily problems and state of mind.

This was an aha moment for me, directing me to the importance of narrowing my focus. It guided me to my current mission of lifting up physicians and healthcare providers who serve.

Tasked as such, I've thought many times about my struggle to fight burnout and find joy when it seemed like a battle, often a daily one. One that I was not winning, one that others were not winning either. Since then I've used a battle theme to address the topic.

Like many battles, there are several strategies that can be successful, and we will discuss a number of them in part 2. In this chapter and the next, we are going to put on our suit of armor, which is critical to ensure victory. We will then fortify the homeland to fend off incoming forces. We will train to become better fighters. We will rethink the battle. Later in part 4, we will finish strong by developing the mind and heart of a warrior.

Donning armor. Fortifying. Training. Rethinking. Developing. Five important battle strategies in order to be successful in our journey to fight burnout and to find joy as a physician.

Put On Your Suit of Armor

Putting on your suit of armor is developing the inner strength, the qualities, and the fortitude to take on the battle—it's a journey. There are a number of ways to do so, so let's get started.

Purpose

The most important way to put on your suit of armor to fight burnout and find joy each day is to know your purpose, to know your why. Understand what you're here on this earth to accomplish. Healthcare providers were given gifts and talents to help others. I believe that we were given that left brain and right brain to serve.

It's interesting that people who serve the community often wear uniforms. Did you know that the three-quarters-length white lab coat in the early 1900s was adopted by physicians from the laboratory to give themselves scientific credibility, as otherwise they were looked upon as a bunch of quacks giving out potions and pills? Ever since, the white lab coat is viewed as a symbol of a scientific healer.

To my fellow physicians and providers, that three-quarters-length white lab coat is your suit of armor. It's your purpose, it's your why. It's why you're different. Each and every day that you put it on, look up to God or higher power, or look inward for strength, straighten your shoulders, and be proud of yourself. You've been asked to serve, you've been asked to sacrifice, you've been asked to reach beyond yourself for the purpose of helping others. And I believe that only the best are given that privilege.

Perhaps you've read the books of Rick Warren, author of *The Purpose Driven Life*; if not I recommend it. His words are truly life-giving. He often says that a life without a purpose is a life not worth living. As I get older, I think about that a lot, and quite frankly, it may explain why I write.

Your purpose guides you to live a more meaningful and fulfilled life. It's the foundation on which you base your thoughts, feelings, decisions, and actions. It fuels your passion, keeps you focused, and increases your productivity.

Accepting responsibility that the health of others depends on you invigorates and rewards. It equips you to better accept the stress of work. It enables you to resist fear. Knowing and living your why promotes joy and gratitude. And as we'll speak to, it gives you the basis on which to define your mountaintop, your place of meaning and finishing strong. Realizing your purpose is critical in fighting burnout and finding joy. So put on your suit of armor—that white coat—and live your purpose.

People Who Serve
Finishing up a consultation with a middle-aged patient, my eyes were drawn to the detective badge strung from a lanyard around his neck. Curious, I asked, "So what's it like to be a detective?"

He responded, "Well, doc, let me put it to you this way. My hours suck. My pay sucks. And people suck. But it's what I do, and I'm glad I do it."

Immediately engaged, I encouraged him to tell me more. Detective Humphrey's primary responsibility was large corporate burglary and theft, substantial crimes that generally dealt with a lot of money. But he actually pointed to one of his simpler crime cases.

A poor elderly woman's home had been burglarized, stripped almost entirely clean of her possessions. But having lost most of her worldly goods, she was most distraught over losing the locket her husband had given to her the day her daughter was born. "Doc, the day I gave her back that locket and saw that joy on her face—that's why I do my job."

We immediately bonded. Every time he comes in now, we smile, exchange a high five, and sit for a few moments to chat. We talk about the battles we fight, the struggles we have, and the common ground we share. Both of us are called to serve and to help others. But both of us struggle with the difficulties associated with the role.

Whether you're a teacher, police officer, firefighter, in the military, or a healthcare professional, you've been called to use your gifts and talents to help others.

Think about how vital it is that you do your job well as a healthcare provider. That you stay healthy, fight the fight, and sacrifice for others. That you identify with the next person you help. That you think about their concerns, their hopefulness, their reliance on you. You're standing in some pretty big shoes and so many patients are counting on you, your compassion, your love. They're counting on your excellence.

If you don't realize and accept this noble responsibility, then finding joy and fulfillment in your work may be difficult. Without the realization and acceptance that this job fulfills a deep need in the community, medicine will just be a job, not a calling. It will be a paycheck, not a meaningful journey.

The daily acceptance of your purpose is the cornerstone of what you do. Your purpose makes you get up every morning to fight the battle and be a great warrior. It's what makes you indispensable, and why the health and well-being of a great nation rests on your shoulders. And to those who accept, the rewards are great.

The origin of your purpose might be different from others. Ever since I was a young boy, I yearned to be a physician. There was no other path that I wished to follow. Looking back now, as a Christian, I believe that God specifically chose me for this role. But like any journey, whether your purpose originates from a transcendent source, an inner strength, or somewhere else, I believe that it guides and motivates each of us to successfully navigate our path and continue to help others. It guides me. It guides you. It guides Detective Humphrey.

Gratefulness

I recently saw a patient I'll call Susan. Her surgery had gone well, and this was to be her last postoperative visit. Attractive, vibrant, looking young for her age, I asked her what she did in retirement to keep busy.

She and her husband were avid travelers. Every month they'd been out on the road, visiting state after state. But since his stroke, her husband's health had severely limited his mobility. Day after day, he sits in his chair. He doesn't want to do things or go places, he just sits. He planted a small tree for Christmas, a family tradition, but it took him nearly all day to accomplish the task, in spite of its small size. Still, it was a big accomplishment under the circumstances of his physical condition. "It's so sad to see him this way," she said.

And following a gentle hug, I remember her looking at me and with a warm smile, saying, "I'm still so grateful just to have him, Dr. MacDiarmid, just so grateful."

The second important way to put on your suit of armor to find joy and fight burnout is to be grateful. I think being grateful is why I can be highly functional and battle my tendencies toward burnout.

I'm so grateful for my beautiful wife Andrea, my daughter Lindsey, and my little dog Maddie. I'm so grateful for my friends back in Canada and in this country. I'm so grateful to be on my end of the stethoscope and not the other. And yes, I'm so grateful to be a physician and to be given the skills and desire to practice my subspecialty.

Experts claim that gratefulness is the antidote to bitterness and resentment, and I believe they're right. Your thoughts control your emotions, which in turn control your behavior. Just sitting and making a list of things to be grateful for a few moments every day can immediately reset negative thinking and get you moving in the right direction again.

Practicing gratitude gives you a healthy big-picture perspective. It takes you off the field where the battle's being fought and places you in the bleachers, shielding you from direct hand-to-hand combat.

From the bleachers, you'll have a much better perspective of the battle. You become less reactive, limiting negative comments and actions. You'll resist the temptation to dwell on the negatives or to get up on your soapbox, which can waste so much energy, time, and emotion. Sitting back, you get a view of the entire story, are more appreciative, and are better able to strategize.

It's in the bleachers where you find joy and fulfillment, even when the fight on the field intensifies. And others around you can benefit too. **Viewing the world with gratefulness will arm you with perspective and wisdom that will be life changing.**

Learn to be Grateful

For many, being grateful doesn't come naturally. Like any skill, we must learn and practice to be so. Buddhism teaches you to be grateful, and that gratitude is cultivated as a habit and is independent of conditions. "Gratitude turns what we have into enough," wrote Melody Beattie. Let me suggest three strategies to develop gratefulness.

The first step in being grateful is to stop taking for granted all the wonderful people, possessions, and circumstances in your life. Take active measure of the gifts and blessings that surround you. Taking anything for granted is the enemy of gratefulness.

Think about your family and friends, your health, that glass of wine you had on Friday, the roof over your head. Think about practicing medicine and the opportunities in life that it's brought you.

I think many are so busy pursuing unmet wants that we don't think about, enjoy, and appreciate what we already have. The pace and busyness of life often can distract us to the point of taking things for granted. Slowing down and developing gratefulness is a big step forward in becoming joyful.

Gratefulness is a choice, like many other emotional states, and practicing being grateful strengthens these patterns of positive thought. Many recommend a few minutes of mindful or verbal rehearsal each morning before the battle begins, or as a recharge at day's end.

Another suggestion, think about the patients you cared for today and place yourself in their shoes. Think of some of the less fortunate ones. Pause and take stock. You'll soon realize that taking things for granted is not a good strategy. You'll immediately feel grateful. Let's face it—we're just one accident, diagnosis, or financial setback away from our life being changed forever.

The second step is to become that "bright side" guy in the bleachers. That sometimes-annoying fan wearing those rose-colored glasses and is always looking at the brighter side of most circumstances. Just when you want to unload, scream, and be affirmed by drawing others into your misery, this person relentlessly bridges the situation to one of positivity. Admit it, just their smile grates on us when we want to be miserable.

I think some use this glass-half-full posture as a smokescreen to deny or to shirk responsibility for problems, sometimes big problems. I know people who are experts at this, and I do not recommend adopting this technique.

But positivity in combination with the perspective achieved when sitting in the bleachers is a powerful mindset to foster joy and fulfillment. Regularly softening the stressors and worries in life with the words "but on the bright side" will help condition you to be grateful. Trust me, it works.

The third way to learn to be grateful is to believe that life's tribulations are opportunities for you to grow and mature. Opportunities to better yourself and to become wiser. It's what faith teaches. It's what we teach and hope for our children. "Failure is the opportunity to begin again, this time more intelligently," Henry Ford said.

I believe that we're tested in areas of our weakness, so we can become more patient, forgiving, and caring. And medicine is quite a testing ground, with seeing thirty patients a day and all those phone calls. The daily bombardment of patient questions and requests, especially those tasked to me by triage, has taught me patience. Patience at work, but also patience at home and in the community. I'm a slow learner to becoming patient, but I'm getting there.

Being grateful for your circumstances, and yes, even the negative ones, is a wonderful lens through which to view the world. I encourage you to sit up in the bleachers and view the daily battle of life play out on the field. As a spectator, give some thought as to how some of the tribulations in your life have bettered you. I'm betting that you have a lot to be grateful for as well.

The perspective of gratefulness is liberating. Learning to be grateful is life-giving. Get off the field of the day-to-day combat and sit back in the bleachers and be grateful.

And if you don't believe me, just ask Susan. Good luck, Susan. Your husband is so fortunate to have you.

The Spirit of Forgiveness

The third way to put on your suit of armor is to live life with a forgiving spirit.

My partners know that I struggle with forgiveness, especially when stressed and fatigued. I get myself in knots much too easily, my thoughts driving my emotions. Whether it's a rude patient, someone who dumped a consult on me, or when things are just not going my way, I can get upset and stew—*for hours*. Worse, I'll wake up in the middle of the night stewing again, flipping back and forth like a fish out of water, reliving the conflict over and over. Ruminating—what a waste of time and energy. It's so unproductive and destructive to myself and to others around me.

And we all know that the person that you or I might be upset with often has no clue about the turmoil that we're experiencing, and likely doesn't care.

Forgiveness is the foundation of a personal and loving relationship. In many circumstances, it occurs naturally as a manifestation of trust and love. In a crisis, a relationship will often never be the same until the one who feels victimized chooses to gracefully forgive the other.

But the same grace and conscious decision to forgive friends and loved ones also rebuilds bridges and brings joy and peace in the workplace. I suspect many work issues that continue to plague me stem from my inability to practice what I preach.

Live life with a forgiving spirit. Forgiveness is the right thing to do. **But**

importantly, forgiveness will liberate your soul. It will lift your burden. It will expand your heart to allow warmth, healing, and growth to inspire your life.

Don't forget about yourself, either. Yes, the most important person in your life for you to forgive is yourself. As we will discuss later, self-forgiveness and the unpacking of one's own baggage is one of the stepping stones to living joyfully.

Forgiveness is a Choice
The choice to forgive begins in your heart. It's a voluntary release of anger, bitterness, or a grudge. While forgiveness is a decision, it's not necessarily an automatic healer of emotions. It helps, but emotions heal over time.

Take an actionable step.

Think of three people in your life who have really hurt or upset you. Your self-centered boss. A dishonest partner or coworker. A patient or person who was rude to you. Someone from years gone by—the one that your initial thought to forgive is, "Absolutely no way. Not going to happen. They don't deserve it. You have no idea what I'm dealing with."

Be radical. Armed by faith or inspired from within, choose to forgive one of them. And I mean truly forgive. Don't listen to "can't." Say no to stubbornness and fear. First think it, then speak it. Purposely verbalize it several times. If appropriate, speak to the person directly. Just do it. And preferably start with someone at work where you're experiencing burnout.

Then, in a month or two, consider how that one decision has impacted your thoughts, your emotions, your words, and your actions. Even though the person's behavior may have remained unchanged, you actually may be feeling better.

If you're feeling more positive, then choose one of the other two people on your list and forgive them. Remember, the deeper the wound, the harder it is to forgive, the greater the potential for healing. When forgiveness defeats "can't," you will be blessed by freedom and joy.

My friend, live life with a forgiving spirit.

Carpe Diem

"Gather ye rosebuds while ye may, old time is still a flying. And this same flower that smiles today, tomorrow will be dying. Gather ye rosebuds while ye may," wrote poet Robert Herrick. The Latin term for that sentiment is *carpe diem*: "seize the day."

"Seize the day. We are food for worms, lads. Because each and every one of us in this room is one day going to stop breathing, turn cold, and die."

I love that scene from *Dead Poets Society*, the 1989 film starring Robin Williams. Set in 1959 at the fictional elite Vermont boarding school Welton Academy, it tells the story of an English teacher, John Keating, who inspires his students through his unorthodox teaching of poetry.

He encourages his students to "make your lives extraordinary," a sentiment he summarizes as carpe diem.

Very few jobs enable one to seize the day like the practice of medicine. Yes, we help. Yes, we reduce pain and suffering. The intimacy of the patient-physician relationship is sacred. It provides fertile ground to carpe diem. Trust, dependence, fear, caring, concern, love—there are so many powerful emotions intermingling so quickly between strangers.

To my fellow physicians: seize the day with compassion. Seize the day by humanizing your patients. Use the intimacy of the patient-physician relationship to impact another far beyond the medical care you provide.

I challenge you to pick one or more patients each day to humanize. Push your interaction beyond the simple actions of writing a prescription, explaining the disease process, or recommending surgery. Sit for a few moments and get to know them. Let them feel like a human being and not just a patient. Ask them what is important in their life. Be compassionate, be all in. Make them smile, make them feel safe, let them know that you've got them covered.

Turn those robotic and often stressful patient care interactions into joyful moments. Not only for them, but for yourself. When you humanize someone, they will humanize you. When you show care and compassion, your heart warms. You will reignite joy and love in your work. The more you do it, the more it will be a part of your every interaction. The spark ignites and spreads quickly.

Perhaps some time later, that same patient may think of the time when they were most afraid and vulnerable, when the care they received reached far beyond the treatment of their medical condition. And in turn, they may share the same grace with others. The same grace when multiplied, would be life- and world-changing.

To my fellow physicians and to those who serve, put on your suit of armor.

- Know your purpose. Know your why.
- Learn to be grateful.
- Live life with a forgiving spirit.
- And "gather ye rosebuds while ye may, old time is still a flying. And this same flower that smiles today, tomorrow will be dying." Yes, carpe diem. Seize the day.

TEAM TALK

Putting on your suit of armor applies to everyone who serves, including nurses and APPs. The battle on the front lines of healthcare is intense, and without donning armor, too many casualties will be realized.

Living your purpose by using your gifts and talents to help others will grant you a meaningful and fulfilled life—a true blessing sought by many, but only experienced by a few.

Learning to be grateful and choosing to forgive will reward you with a tremendous treasure.

Loving and humanizing others will empower you to seize the day as you compassionately care for and lift up our nation.

To all providers, put on your suit of armor and let's go to battle together.

A Journey Moment

A great warrior needs a suit of armor that sustains and protects. Any weakness in it can threaten one's joy. Digging deep into the following questions will help you strengthen your armor.

What is your purpose as a healthcare provider? Do you believe that your purpose benefits others? If yes, is helping others satisfying and fulfilling?

_____

_____

_____

_____

_____

_____

_____

Are you grateful to be a physician or do you tend to take being one for granted? Why are you grateful?

_____

_____

_____

_____

_____

_____

_____

Is there someone at work that you need to forgive? Are you willing to be radical and forgive them now? Write down that you have forgiven that person and rehearse your words over and over.

_____

_____

_____

_____

_____

_____

_____

In the midst of a busy workday, do you take time to humanize patients? If no, decide to do so this week, and at week's end, journal your experience. This space is waiting for you . . . see you in a week.

_____

_____

_____

_____

_____

_____

_____

CHAPTER 8

MOUNTAINTOP DECISIONS

I was probably in my third year of premed when I spent the summer employed as an ambulance attendant and orderly at our local hospital in eastern Canada. During work, I received a call from my parents informing me that my grandmother was ill and in the hospital. I ran to the emergency department as quickly as I could, and witnessed my Nanny in code blue. As an orderly, I had seen a few codes; some people were saved, and some did not survive. But this one was different: my grandmother had been rushed in, likely in heart failure. And in her late eighties, only frail because of her age, it was her time to be the one who didn't come back. I think of the tube between her lips, the stillness of her hospital gown partially covering her petite arms, each with an intravenous. I think of her lovely and delicate self. Oddly, in the midst of the organized chaos, her passing seemed peaceful.

Years later, when I was working in a small community as an emergency room physician, a patient had taken his own life by putting a gun to his head and somehow pulled the trigger. Thinking back on it now, it was the furthest thing imaginable from a peaceful passing.

The calm I experienced during Nanny's death was because I knew the loving and peaceful life she'd chosen to live. A calm, beautiful existence that she chose not only for herself, but to share with family, friends, and with others. Not knowing the suicidal man or his circumstances, I can't imagine what he must have been going through to end his own life. How hopeless, sad, or desperate he must have been. In the midst of his tragedy, I wonder if he had made a number of life decisions that were less desirable and affirming.

Given these two different scenarios of lives ending, I want to share with you a final way to put on your suit of armor. It's a life-giving choice that I encourage you to make each and every day. A decision that will help you find joy and fight burnout. It's a simple recommendation that can inspire and encourage, especially if you're tending toward or fighting burnout.

Make Mountaintop Decisions

The fifth and arguably the most important or actionable way to put on your suit of armor is to make mountaintop decisions and—hear me loud and clear—to make them several times daily.

In the deepest of contrasts to the valley, the mountaintop is that sacred place where you find joy, peace, virtue, and contentment. It's where you realize your purpose. The summit is that meaningful place in life where you know that all the negatives and stresses associated with the practice of medicine are worth it. It's when you live in the moment. You're fully engaged, you're all in.

It's a transcendent place enriched by feelings of gratitude and forgiveness. It's where you seize the day. Most importantly, it's where you stand and look back over your life, you look out over those valleys, and you say to yourself "job well done." Those magical words of finishing strong.

So how do we find our mountaintop? How do we pursue a life with meaning and finishing strong?

It comes down to a decision and a choice. The decision is to take ownership and accept the realities of the world of medicine in which we now live. Yes, we are commoditized, yes we are stressed and devalued, yes electronic medical records are killing us. But in order to reach our mountaintop, we need to accept all of this—because let's face it, the good old days of healthcare are over.

And then there's the choice. What I've learned in my personal struggle to fight burnout and to find joy is that regularly I find myself at a crossroads: Will I choose to continue to walk the downward path into the valley of frustration, self-pity, bitterness, and resentment? The path into the valley that so negatively affects my joy, my career, my patient-physician relationships, my friendships, and yes, even my home life? Or do I choose to follow the steep and difficult upward path onto the mountaintop of virtue and meaning? A path so steep that I believe some will only be able to ascend by one of two ways.

For many, they will be pushed up by their fear of living in the valley and its adverse effects on themselves and others around them. Fear is a great motivator. Put your fear behind you and allow it to push you up toward the mountaintop. Looking back on my struggles, it's what initially motivated me.

I'm confident that many will be pulled up to their mountaintop by their inner strength, or perhaps their transcendent strength, and their realization that they exist on this earth to use their gifts and talents to help others and to serve. And they're willing to accept the circumstances and challenges of the difficult climb in order to achieve their goal.

To my fellow physicians, please make it your ritual to make mountaintop decisions, to make them several times daily, and choose to follow the upward path to the summit.

So what does this look like? Start thinking, saying, and doing things that align yourself with living on your mountaintop. Cheerlead and empower your staff. Take a few extra moments to laugh with a patient. Speak with your partner about an issue rather than burying it. Leave work at work, and be the spouse, parent, child, and friend the people in your life deserve.

And stop thinking, saying, and doing the things you know are not good for you and are dragging you down into the valley. Don't stand up on your soapbox in the physician's lounge, make sarcastic remarks to the scrub nurse, stew over that rude patient or manipulative partner, and go home angry and bark at your daughter. And for some, don't consume too much alcohol and binge angrily in front of inflammatory news shows.

Fist Pumps

It's important to reward yourself. On a daily basis, I enjoy a triumphant fist pump each time I make a mountaintop decision. These decisions might be thinking, saying, or doing something positive, but more often by *not* thinking, saying, or doing something negative. And it feels great.

Yes, give yourself a fist pump. It's a gesture of triumph or affirmation in which the forearm is raised with fist clenched, then swung downward in a vigorous pumping motion. A celebratory gesture so commonly used by athletes and millions of others worldwide. There's just something about it that makes you feel great. It's encouraging. It's uplifting.

Most often, at the end of my workday, I'll take stock. I call this "base camp," where I think about what I did well, what things I didn't do so well and need improvement, and yes, the things I really messed up and need to do my best to avoid in the future. Base camp is a great time for personal growth and reflection.

This simple fist pump exercise can actually condition you to act, speak, and even think differently. It conditions you to start anticipating stressors and circumstances, and you begin making mountaintop decisions proactively.

I fist pump before entering the doctor's lounge, committing to avoid negative discussions about the state of healthcare. I fist pump pulling into the driveway at home, when I decide to abandon listing my daily complaints to my family, and instead celebrate the day with a smile and life-affirming hug. Every day, countless fist pumps.

Once you start implementing this simple behavioral exercise, you start getting your old self back. You start catching yourself smiling more, being less reactive and cynical, and actually lifting up those around you.

Start small. Start with opportunities within your circle of influence, within your circle of friends. But don't underestimate the power of the compound effect of incremental success or action over time. Make mountaintop decisions, and enjoy the fist pumps.

I hope and pray that thousands of providers nationwide will regularly celebrate with a congratulatory fist pump as they live their journey loving and caring for our nation. **Yes, please join the Fist Pumps Revolution and begin the journey to your mountaintop now!**

Valleys or Mountaintops?

I think the mountaintop is the place where Nanny finished. For decades when I visited her, she sat in a beautifully embroidered, almost majestic antique chair. She was always smiling and listening. She loved watching us eat her freshly baked cookies and the apple pie that she prepared just for us. She chose to be content. She knew her purpose, and she always seemed to be at peace. I believe that she regularly made choices aligning herself with her mountaintop. And I think at the end, she knew where she was going. I'd wager that she would have said that she finished strong. She was on her summit.

Though I didn't know him, I suppose it's fair to assume that the man who took his own life was living in the deepest of valleys. Perhaps in his words, he might have called it hell. A deep descent into a valley possibly impacted by unhealthy decisions and choices. So sad. So destructive.

So, in closing, let me leave you with a question.

Is it better to live with:
Resentment or gratefulness?
Anger or forgiveness?
Survival or carpe diem?
Burnout or purpose and meaning?

Or perhaps, more simply put, valleys or mountaintops?

TEAM TALK

Making mountaintop decisions and choosing to follow the right path is a life-giving journey for nurses and APPs.

The daily crossroads will come quickly and will be never-ending. Whether it's a patient's difficult family, learning that a coworker shirked their responsibility, the never-satisfied supervisor, the poorly functioning EMR program, and many other challenges, these will be regular crossroads in which you get to choose how you will respond.

You get to choose what you will think, say, and do with each decision that either lifts you up to the summit or drags you down into the valley of burnout.

Make it your daily ritual to make mountaintop decisions. Don't forget base camp, and yes, enjoy those congratulatory fist pumps.

A JOURNEY MOMENT

I would like to leave you with three things to work on in making your own mountaintop decisions, three actionable steps. (You may need an additional journal to accomplish this task.)

First, define your mountaintop. Define it in terms of your work, family, friends, community, and your spiritual, mental, and physical health. Give it a lot of thought. Think about what decisions and actions would make you more joyful and fulfilled. Don't try to complete the exercise during one sitting; expect rewrites and revisions. Consider discussing it with loved ones and colleagues or mentors.

Second, envision your valley and what that valley looks like in any of your domains. Be honest with yourself, be specific, and write it down. Then reflect how each valley might look like in five years if you continue on the same path. Ask yourself—is that really what you want? Is that really how you want to live and finish? Remember, fear is a great motivator.

Finally, take ownership and accept the situation you currently find yourself in as a healthcare provider, as a friend, as a member of your family and community. Accept your current spiritual, mental, and physical health. And then, take action.

As a start, list three mountaintop decisions that you'll make this week. Stop thinking, saying, and doing things that are bad for you. And start thinking, saying, and doing things that are good and align you with your mountaintop. And don't forget the fist pumps.

For example, if you walk into the physician's lounge and realize that they're in the midst of a heated and emotional discussion about the woeful state of healthcare, say nothing. Have your salad, your favorite beverage, but don't engage. And when you leave to head back to work, look up with a fist pump. You deserve it.

When you arrive home at day's end, still angry and frustrated with your partner or administrator, resist the temptation to unload on your family. Trade complaining for a smile, and take a walk with your loved one. And look up— fist pump.

And if you're having a really rough day, perhaps not even sure if you can make it or continue, and your frustration is palpable, go into your office and shut the door. Sit down and bow your head.

Ask yourself, What am I here for? What purpose in my life am I here to fulfill? And when you figure that out, look up with a fist pump. Then open that door, and get back to the battle. There are too many people on the other side of that door counting on you for you to get stuck on your frustrations.

Start slow. Take baby steps up the path to the summit. Then next week, list three more mountaintop decisions. Keep on doing so until you find yourself making positive progress spontaneously. Yes, until you are making mountaintop decisions automatically.

Accept the short-term failures, the slips and falls. Trust me, there will be plenty. But get back up and keep on climbing. Some days the climb will be easy, some days difficult, others might feel impossible. But keep going. Finish on the summit; finish strong.

And as you climb to the summit, whether the load that day is light or heavy, remember that you have on your suit of armor. That three-quarters-length white lab coat is why you're different. It's why you are a great climber and that you'll be successful in reaching your mountaintop. When you put on your lab coat each morning, look up to God or higher power, or look inward for strength, straighten your shoulders, and be proud of yourself.

You've been asked to serve, you've been asked to sacrifice, you've been asked to reach beyond yourself, for others. And I believe that only the best are given that privilege.

Define your mountaintop:

Work:

_____

_____

_____

_____

Family:

_____

_____

_____

_____

Friends:

_____

_____

_____

_____

Community:

_____

_____

_____

_____

Health:

_____

_____

_____

_____

What is your valley?

Work:

_____

_____

_____

Family:

_____

_____

_____

Friends:

_____

_____

_____

_____

Community:

_____

_____

_____

_____

Health:

_____

_____

_____

_____

Take action:

List three mountaintop decisions. (Week 1)

1. _____
2. _____
3. _____

List three mountaintop decisions. (Week 2)

1. _____
2. _____
3. _____

List three mountaintop decisions. (Week 3)

1. _____
2. _____
3. _____

CHAPTER 9

FORTIFY THE HOMELAND: LEADERSHIP, VISION, SAFETY, AND EMPOWERMENT

In order to find joy and fight burnout, you're going to have to fortify the homeland. Fortifying the homeland is necessary to ward off the attack from external forces.

You need to build a workplace that inspires you to go to work in the morning, makes you feel safe when you're there, and when you go home at night you feel a sense of fulfillment.

We need to do this because the opposite is destructive. If your perception of your work environment is one of death by a thousand cuts, or perhaps one of resentment and frustration, it's going to destroy you much faster that all those external forces that you might be blaming. In addition, when you're already weakened from within your own homeland, your ability to fight off outside enemies is jeopardized.

I think that dysfunctional homelands are much more common than not, and that many physicians' feelings of frustration and joylessness are related to their daily experiences within their workplace. Interpersonal work dynamics are a difficult business and physicians are not immune to this. In fact, the stress in a medical office might amplify the problems. But there are numerous opportunities to make things better.

Remember that the positive things you think, say, and do, and the negative things you don't think, say, and do in fortifying the homeland aligns you with

75

your mountaintop. It aligns you with joy and meaning, giving you more fist pump opportunities.

Don't underestimate the positive impact of making small homeland improvements. One by one, you can make a difference. In fortifying the homeland, we'll explore decisions and mindsets and offer a number of pragmatic suggestions that will help you find greater happiness. Although some of this may be applied more to private practicing physicians, many thoughts can be applied to those who are hospital employed. I've also dedicated an entire section later that addresses fortification for employed providers.

I challenge you to read this section, reread it, and then begin a journey. Plan how you might positively impact your workplace and fortify your homeland. **The goal: make work a no burnout zone.**

Leadership

So, what does a fortified homeland and workplace look like? First, it's led by a physician leader. It's not led by an administrator. It's not led by groupthink.

A workplace should be led by an all-in leader who has the time, energy, and fortitude to sacrifice for others. A leader who can make tough decisions and keep everyone accountable, including himself or herself. A leader who fosters healthy communication in which everyone is heard. Listening, mutual respect, and trust keep a homeland fortified.

The need for strong leadership is constant. I believe that leadership occurs at multiple levels, yet certainly rests on the shoulders of each physician. Within our own circle of influence, our steadfast commitment to leading our staff and those around us is so impactful. And when successful, leads to more joy and less burnout.

Ask yourself: How am I leading? **Identify one thing you can do tomorrow at work to lead your staff to a better place. Maybe that can be just asking someone's opinion who may not usually have a voice, and really listen.**

Lofty Vision
The leaders of a fortified homeland have a lofty vision. I believe that the lofty vision is to provide a work environment that nourishes and brings joy and fulfillment to those who serve. An environment that inspires its providers and staff to live on their mountaintop, to live out their why. A work environment should encourage patient-centric excellence and support providers and staff to use their gifts and talents to help others.

When your staff shares this lofty vision and they believe in what you believe, the harmony provided brings happiness, excellence, and less burnout to all. Your patients will also love their wonderful care.

Many of your staff and coworkers choose to work in healthcare for reasons similar to yours. They want to help others. They want to serve. They want to be nourished and inspired. When that is the case, they won't even consider switching to a new employer whose vision differs for a few extra dollars. Loyalty prevails when the vision is clear and unified.

I encourage you to speak out, and more importantly, to live out your lofty vision daily. Provide a work environment that inspires and encourages those around you. Be a model to your staff that patient-centric excellence matters. Battle your stress, your fatigue, those frustrating days, and continue to live in excellence. It's worth it.

Safe
A fortified homeland is safe.

One of the biggest tragedies of the American healthcare system is the indoctrination of the culture of Wall Street and corporations into our hospitals, in which you sacrifice your employees for multi-million-dollar profits and the fiduciary responsibility is to the shareholder. That does not make an employee feel safe. And now hospital systems are showing multi-million-dollar spreadsheets and met metrics to a board of directors and many administrators are making millions.

What's happened in hospitals is that the people actually providing the care—the doctors, nurses, and other providers—are not being cared for. In fact, in many cases they're being sacrificed for profit. That environment breeds apathy and mediocrity, it breeds an every-man-for-himself type of attitude, it breeds a lack of excellence, and it fuels burnout.

This apathy results in patients sitting in their own urine or stool for an hour with their call light on, desperate for assistance, because the hospital is understaffed. When administrators hire too many inexperienced nurses in order to save money, a catheter balloon ends up being blown up in a man's urethra much too often. It looks like a lack of continuity of care when one hospitalist inadequately signs off to another. And it looks like medical errors and accidental deaths because giant healthcare systems are profiting millions from understaffing and hiring poorly skilled providers, and yet still marketing "world-class care" to their communities.

For those of you in private practice: do not run your practice this way. Unlike healthcare systems, you're not too big to fail.

Value your staff, and most importantly, make them feel safe. Provide them safety in their employment, fair compensation, safety in airing their voices, and safety in their interactions with patients. Trust is priceless. As is the case in any intimate relationship, once trust is lost, it's very difficult to earn back.

Your staff need to feel like valuable members of the healthcare team. They want to be respected and feel important. They want to use their gifts and ideas to make a difference. If your staff are reduced to numbers on a payroll, you will never inspire joy. Respect and value each employee for who they are as a person, and you will inspire loyalty.

When your staff know that you have their backs, they will give their hearts and souls to the practice, to the patients, and to you. Once again there will be more excellence, more joy, and less burnout. Fist pump.

So, Do Your Staff Feel Safe?

Think about this before answering. Denial might prevent you from admitting that your staff do not feel as safe as you might think—this will only lead you to a more dysfunctional homeland. It will only promote less excellence and more burnout.

The high turnover of staff and nurses in hospitals and practices, I believe, is largely due to them not feeling safe. They don't trust their employers or share a common vision with them. Too many feel like a replaceable cog in a wheel, and loyalty disappears once a person is commoditized. They feel like an assembly line worker who can be easily replaced. They, too, were called to this profession; it's sad to waste such a wonderful and caring soul.

Empowerment

Most afternoons, I stop by the hospital physician lunchroom and grab a quick salad or soup of the day. The chicken is reasonable, the meatballs are good, the food overall gets a passing grade, and I appreciate it.

John's primary responsibility is making sure the buffet-style physician breakfast, lunch, and all the snacks and drinks are set out. John has worked there for nearly a decade, and what he does and how he does it is perfect. The counters are kept perfectly clean. The food is always restocked. He gives you a smile that lights up the room with peace, gratitude, and giving. If I had a dollar for every time he has asked me if lunch was good, always offering to run to the kitchen for a secret something if I needed or wanted it, I'd be rich. He makes me feel special and valued.

Just yesterday at lunch, I asked John what makes him tick. What makes him do such a good job day after day?

With humility, John softly responded with a smile, "Doc, I just like to be excellent."

But with further prodding, John added, "I've always been that way; it's important to me. It's how my mom raised me and my brothers and sisters."

A Generational Gift

More and more, it seems, we're living in a culture of what I refer to as "an assembly line robotic mentality." One in which people go to work not understanding the importance of their job, not interested in the task at hand, and not caring very much about it. For many, it's a paycheck and that's it.

It saddens me that this culture of not caring has become so pervasive, especially in the healthcare profession. The patients, the physicians, the employer, the nurses, and the staff—yes, everyone—lose. The more we corporatize and depersonalize the business of healthcare and hire lower paid and less qualified nurses and staff while the system prioritizes profit, this problem is just going to get worse.

A partial remedy to this problem is empowerment.

In a perfect world, everyone would be self-motivated like John. But failure is everywhere. Good or bad, that leaves some of the responsibility of making a positive impact and changing behavior to employers, like you and me.

I encourage you to empower and train your staff to use their gifts to help others. Empower them to make independent decisions and to take responsibility. Affirm, cheerlead, and applaud. Such verbal recognition lifts up many and is much more effective than criticism.

Let your nurses and staff fail. Trust me, they will. But lift them up, retrain, and encourage. Pull them up toward excellence. Pull them forward toward their mountaintop.

By doing so, you'll uncover their pride and self-confidence. You'll uncover a confident soul who helps both you and your patients. Those with confidence look out for one another, it's not every man for themselves. One of our nurses struggled early in her career from lack of experience and confidence. She had difficulty accomplishing tasks and was always worried about doing something wrong. With some training, cheerleading, and encouragement from physicians and teammates, she is now one of our top providers. **Empowered staff will reduce your burden, reduce your stress, and reduce your burnout.** Fist pump.

Please invest time, your caring, and resources in your nurses and staff. You may be one of the few employers ever to do so. Don't underestimate the greater good you'll provide by empowering others to reach their true potential. A potential that, without your empowerment, might never be realized.

Most people, when empowered and encouraged, become more dependable, hard-working, happier, and fulfilled at home, in their community, and in their life. In return they are more likely to raise and empower the next generation to be so enabled. Like John, his siblings, and his mom. Empowerment is a beautiful and generational gift.

Not only does John drive excellence at our hospital, but he is also an accomplished and gifted musician and drummer. His band regularly rocks it out in Greensboro and throughout the Carolinas.

Cheers to you, John. Thanks for rocking. Thanks for being you.

TEAM TALK

Nurses and APPs must fortify the homeland to help ward off external forces that may be threatening their joy and causing burnout. As an employed provider, narrow your focus and energy to the homeland where you can most readily influence and positively impact.

All providers are leaders by looking after and caring for the person next to them. Within your circle of influence, listen to, respect, and help your fellow coworker, and assist them whenever possible. Your workplace, yourself, and the world around you will forever benefit.

Nurses and advanced practice providers also fortify the homeland by helping provide an environment that nourishes and encourages others to serve and deliver patient-centric excellence. They provide safety by helping and covering the backs of one another. They discourage assembly line robotic behavior, both from themselves and from their teammates. They affirm and empower one another to make independent decisions and to use their gifts to help others.

Fortifying the homeland by leading, by living out your lofty vision, by making others feel safe, and by empowering those around you is the responsibility of all. It's a responsibility that brings joy and reduces burnout.

A JOURNEY MOMENT

List at least three ways that you can empower your staff to take responsibility and to make independent decisions. Encourage them and be ready to lift them up when they fail. And in doing so, do you believe that they will feel happier and more fulfilled? Do you believe that this will help fortify the homeland?

1. _____
2. _____
3. _____

Once you have experienced positive results and fruits from your labor as a result of empowering others, consider coming up with three more.

1. _____
2. _____
3. _____

CHAPTER 10

FORTIFY THE HOMELAND: COMMUNICATION, ACCOUNTABILITY, AND COMPENSATION

L eadership, with a lofty vision, provides safety and empowers your staff. These are effective and important strategies in fortifying the homeland. But in our battle against burnout, they're not enough. Let's discuss more ways to shore up the defenses.

Communication

Perhaps one of the biggest challenges and sources of loss of joy and burnout in physician practices is unhealthy communication. Many physicians believe that they're not being listened to and that they have no voice. And in many cases, they're right.

Once kings and queens of their own domain, many physicians feel that they are now controlled by partners and administrators. This dynamic is not only destructive to the organization, but it significantly promotes burnout. I think the problem is worsening as groups continue to expand in size in their attempt to survive.

Many private practices are managed by open discussion and by a majority wins, equal voting process. Seemingly fair, this structure does have its problems. Many highly independent, highly intelligent individuals have an "I'm always right" survival mentality. With a room full of people who all want to get their way, it's commonplace to make poor decisions and be inefficient. At times, conflicts arise. It's a team full of captains; I call it the stumbling democracy.

But is it really democratic? My experience with this is that many intelligent men and women are actually influenced by groupthink. Groupthink controlled by the same two or three individuals who are dominantly vocal. The rest are reluctant to express their own opinions or are even bullied, while others either can't be bothered or are easily swayed. Swayed by the notorious "but what if that happens" or half-truth rationalizations. With meeting agendas predetermined and controlled, the same few run the show.

The results of leadership by groupthink can lead to poor performance as a practice and where no one takes responsibility. Poor outcomes are ignored by physicians and by administration. Functional processes stumble as a result of bad leadership. And from the silenced minority comes frustration, bitterness, and resentment. The famous "I don't know, I just work here" is voiced by many. In many cases, it becomes a group divided.

When conflict divides a group into two camps—no matter the issue—the harmony and function of the homeland is jeopardized. Mutual trust and respect withers. Some physicians leave. Other homelands split, with one group sometimes selling out to the hospital. Interpersonal conflict is a big deal. It's emotional, it's personal.

Often, it's not the actual decisions that cause strife, but the process of not being heard, the perception that voices are oppressed. And it's tough living with the consequences of decisions you didn't agree with after a discussion where you were ignored. In fact, sometimes in this situation, people end up *hoping* that aspects of the organization fail, just for spite.

Let me provide you with a three-step strategy to help you navigate these difficult communication challenges.

First, define the problem.

Really think through the communication issues that are negatively impacting the greater good of the practice. Be as specific as possible and write them down. Concentrate on how decisions are being made, not so much on particular examples and outcomes—there lies too much emotion and conflict.

It's the process that needs to change, and the results will take care of themselves. But it's important to take inherent bias, emotions, and personal conflicts into consideration, all potential enemies of solving difficult issues. Let the truth dictate group discussion. I always have to remind myself that heated negotiations are no time for exaggeration. Avoid amplifying the issue with words like *always* and *never*.

Define the communication problem:

1. _____
2. _____
3. _____
4. _____

Second, look in the mirror and redefine the problem. Ask yourself what role you've played in allowing or enabling the communication breakdown. Were you silent? Did you fear the consequences of standing up and being counted? Did you nod yes just to get along? It's in the mirror that you'll realize that you may be equally culpable.

Agreeableness is a personality trait characterized by compassion, friendliness, politeness, and empathy. People rich in agreeableness put others first. They're good listeners and team players. This is valuable when practicing medicine, but the same individuals may have a hard time saying no, and are potentially more readily controlled by groupthink. But blaming only them, and not yourself, I argue, is a bad strategy. Don't allow agreeableness to breed complacency.

Redefine the problem (your role):

1. _____

2. _____

3. _____

4. _____

Third, it's time to act. Action by voice, by thought, or by feet.

Act by voice. Use your voice, or your voice magnified by a number of others. Stand up and be counted. Especially when you're a lone ranger, such braveness is not for the faint of heart. Be a challenger.

Choose your words wisely. Identify the functional problem and how it's negatively impacting the group. Focus on the dynamic that you're trying to positively impact. Healthier group communication benefits all, and efforts to combat this common good is difficult even for the reluctant groupthinkers.

But whether paralyzed by fear or other, many are unable to speak. Confronting others is difficult and can expose one to harsh criticism. Groupthink craves power and control, and it will not relinquish it easily. Trust me, I get how difficult it is to expose yourself to this power dynamic.

If you choose to be silent, then *act by thought.* By thoughtfully considering your own actions or inaction, you consciously take responsibility and recognize your silent culpability, which gives many a certain degree of peace and acceptance. This thinking will lead to less finger-pointing and reduce anger and stress. Sharing some of the blame oddly is a solution to personal torment. In other occasions, it motivates the silent to finally stand tall and be counted. By thought, you will find a better place to live within the turmoil.

And last, *act by feet.* Like any relationship, sometimes the only solution to the problem is solved by finding another homeland for your skills and patients. With some homelands, the dysfunction cannot be overcome.

Difficult and brave choices of walking are best made slowly, and expectations of greener pastures elsewhere must be guarded. Making that decision is never easy—please be careful in doing so. In the short term, there are often no winners. Change can hurt, but sometimes it is for the better. But your personal and family's long-term happiness and health is priceless. If you have to walk, do it.

Accountability

A fortified homeland has rules. **A fortified homeland has accountability. This is easy to say, but difficult to do and enforce, especially for physicians.**

In our clinic, we have a rule that at least one of our three advanced practice providers must be at work at all times. They must coordinate personal time off in order to accommodate that condition. Their presence is vital in handling patient volume and managing sub-acute work-ins. On a busy day, we need all hands on deck.

Still, as I write this, in the next four days we have no APPs in the house—zero. Without them, it's going to be tough for the on-call physician. This happens repeatedly.

Here's another issue: in our clinic, we have a rule that if a patient shows up more than fifteen minutes late, their appointment needs to be rescheduled. Late patients stress clinic and staff, and providing them care often sacrifices timely care to others.

Still, regularly, tardy patients are checked in and added on to the already full and running-behind schedule. When this occurs, the patients who honored their appointment time have to wait even longer. The cycle adds more stress and frustration to the physicians and staff.

In our clinic, we have a rule that we don't treat bladder infections over the phone. We believe that it affects quality and safety, and the ever-increasing number of requests in recent years is not sustainable. Our triage team offers patients a same-day appointment with an APP, or recommends for them to contact their primary care physician.

Still, our physicians are repeatedly tasked by triage to send in a prescription for a patient who has called in thinking they might have a urinary tract infection. The result: lower quality care, increased provider frustration, and more burnout.

In our clinic, the physicians are equally guilty of not following rules on a regular basis. Asking the resident physician to perform duties that they are not responsible for, not completing surgical scheduling sheets and patient follow-up orders, not unblocking open schedules . . . the list goes on. And arguably, time after time, it seems to be the same perpetrators.

So, What's the Deal?

I'm not trying to throw our clinic, the administrative staff, or my partners and I under the bus, but let's face it: we have a problem. And the problem is we are not obeying our own rules, or not *respecting* the rules that were established to uphold quality care and govern a functional, productive workplace. The problem is also a lack of accountability and leadership. Accountability requires confrontation, and that is not easy or comfortable.

See, without rules and accountability, you have anarchy. Not only does anarchy foster poor outcomes, it erodes the spirit and trust of those who are actually engaged and to whom rules matter.

To the conscientious, allowing others to do what they want without consequence fosters resentment. It fosters lack of respect for the organization, and breeds a "why should I care?" and "every-man-for-themselves" mentality. It fosters a perception that rules apply to some but not others. Anarchy fuels burnout.

You can't have leadership without accountability. The analogy is it's like a ship without a rudder. So many leaders are not true leaders. Just having a position in the hierarchy arguably has no predictive value in one's actual leadership skill. The position of leadership doesn't give you any predictability of their ability and willingness to sacrifice, to empower, to lead, and to keep others accountable.

Most physicians have limited leadership skills and training, and may not really appreciate the value that good leadership brings. In my experience with many administrators, they seem trained in checking the boxes, talking a good game, job preservation for themselves, but not true leadership.

The Solution

Rule #1: Find the right leader.

Understand your organization's needs, its strengths and weaknesses, and list them out. Identify the qualities in a leader that are most important for your organization. Communicate these to the leaders you have now, and if they can't deliver, find new leadership. (Easier said than done.)

Rule #2: The standard is the standard.

I absolutely knew that Rhett was the right person to ask for leadership tutelage. Our friendship grew on the sidelines of the volleyball court, watching our kids play. He's a former Wake Forest lineman, and now runs a car dealership here in Greensboro. I can only imagine the daily pressure and responsibility he faces.

I often stop by his office to chat for a few minutes. I admire Rhett and value our relationship. His character is to the point, no bull, saying things like, "Yes I'm listening," and "Yes I care what you have to say." He's consistent and trusted, respected and liked by his employees.

Having presented to him my topic that rules matter, he immediately responded:

"Scott, around here we have a philosophy. 'The standard is the standard, period!' You buy in and agree to it when hired. We meet and speak to it weekly. We all keep everyone accountable, and I mean everyone. The standard applies not only to outcome, but also to processes and how we function, and how we treat customers and fellow employees."

When I told Rhett about the numerous rules that weren't being followed in our clinic, I asked hypothetically, "So, what would you do when you're tasked by triage to call in a prescription for Mrs. Smith's urinary tract infection?"

He said, "First, I need to understand whether I have a 'doing problem' or a 'knowing problem.' Is it will, or is it skill? Each one, as you can imagine, is handled differently. We ask, we coach, and we retrain the processes and why the standard matters. We encourage and highlight the importance of everyone on the team doing their job, and when necessary, I terminate. The mission is too important."

I chuckled, imagining what Rhett would do working in many physician offices or the hospital. It's a homeland without accountability, and in Rhett's world, is unacceptable.

Rule #3: Give the gift of accountability.

There's no question that one of the greatest things you can give to your employees is the gift of accountability. Being accountable is taking responsibility or ownership for decisions made, actions taken, and assignments completed. Accountable individuals are committed to doing their daily work and accomplishing their goals.

Holding others accountable builds trust and improves morale and performance within the organization. It eliminates time and effort spent on unproductive activities and behavior. It teaches people to value their work and increases team members' skills and confidence.

Empower your staff to take responsibility and to be accountable. Set the expectation that rules matter, and that the standard is the standard, and give them the tools and empower them to reach that expectation. Provide them with the security to admit to mistakes and that it's okay to ask for help.

And watch them grow and develop at work, at home, and in their communities. Fist pump.

Rule #4: Of course there are always exceptions.

I can hear it now: the exceptions argument that torpedoes my "rules matter" philosophy. The people who rationalize an individual event as one where the rules can be overridden because of some unique circumstance or exception, as though it occurs infrequently. But as you can imagine, the issue keeps happening.

My response is polite: that's the problem. They're exactly right, there are *always* exceptions, and unfortunately always means multiple times a week, not once a year. So, the result is anarchy.

On a positive note there is an important takeaway. Yes, there are exceptions. And it's in the exceptions that we empower our staff to grow even further, to mature, and to become more self-confident and highly functioning. We want staff to bend or break rules when they deem necessary. We want them to make independent decisions with the greater good in mind. Yes, the person is late for their appointment and the rules are the rules, but also, that person might have driven from three hours away, out of state. Yes, the person wants a prescription called in and the rules are the rules, but the difference is she's crying on the phone because she can't come into the clinic—she's stuck out of town and really suffering.

It's in the exceptions that we all learn and grow together. Empower your staff such that when they consciously act against a rule for the greater good, the decision is documented, discussed, and used as a team-building opportunity. Especially valuable are the ones when, in retrospect, the decision was less than ideal and can be used as an example of what not to repeat in the future.

Just recently, we had a late patient allowed to check in that severely disrupted the clinic's flow and adversely affected many. My nurses were already stressed but hung in there and shouldered the added burden. Looking back, the front desk staff probably made the wrong call by letting the patient check in, but they were trying to accommodate a frail and elderly patient. Their compassion for her rationalized their exception. Unfortunately, I didn't discuss this with them and lost a valuable teaching and empowering opportunity. Cheers to them for caring and for trying to help!

We need people to think and to make wise and independent decisions. We need excellence and less passing the buck.

Rule #5: Reward the process, not the outcome.
Let's face it. We live in an outcome-based society. In corporate America, and now increasingly in healthcare, success and reward is based on meeting prede-termined goals. How they are attained is becoming less important.

How much did you bill? How many work relative value units did you generate? What was your patient satisfaction score? These are artificial indices propagated within the last ten years, but have grown dominant as both daily measurements of productivity and stressors. And with the targets always moving, the pressure associated with chasing the carrot is smothering.

Blind pursuit of target deliverables can sometimes incentivize inappropriate behavior and foster an every-man-for-themselves mentality. It can disincen-tivize a team culture and promote resentment.

To my fellow physicians—focus rewards instead on the process, especially when it comes to your nurses and staff. Encourage, recognize, and reward integrity, extra effort, and caring. Reward making decisions, helping other employees, and accountability. Reward behavior that represents the philosophy and culture that you're trying to instill. Trust me, the outcomes will take care of themselves.

Reward your administrator. Bonus and incentivize on how well he or she empowers others and develops a culture of accountability. How well they coach and train. How well they model and encourage the clinic's lofty vision. How much they are respected and trusted. An easy measurement is when employee turnover is high, then Houston, you have a problem.

If administration is not up to the task and you're endlessly living in the world of "there are always exceptions," seek new leadership. Think like Rhett and terminate. The health and well-being of yourself, your staff, your patients, and the organization is too valuable to accept any less.

Compensation

I think most of us would agree that financial reward fosters hard work and motivation. We all want to be respected, valued, and importantly, compensated fairly.

But unfortunately, the opposite is often true. Perceived unfair compensation discourages even the most motivated. When you have to take on an extra case or see more patients for little reward, the perception is that the extra effort is no longer worth it.

In fact, my relative income for the same amount of work continues to decline. Working harder and making less year after year adds to physician burnout.

Beyond being discouraging, lower provider income can upset a once healthy group dynamic and destabilize the homeland. There's no question that when the food chain is scarce, the hyenas start fighting. Groups become divided, there's finger-pointing, criticizing, and resenting each other, all because of money.

We all know that there's no perfect compensation plan in a privately-owned physician group. There are always perceived winners and losers. But as physician incomes continue to decline, many of the high producers who see more patients and perform more procedures and surgeries are getting tired of subsidizing others. And they're not happy.

Beware. It's just a matter of time before the high performers slow down and do less. It's human nature. As they regress to the mean, especially in a high fixed overhead model, the overall financial health of the organization can decline significantly.

The result will be that quarterly distributions and incomes decline further. Some providers will then produce even less. The hyenas get hungrier and angrier. Less joy, more stress, and more burnout. I call it the death spiral.

Let's face it. Assuming that each doctor is providing safe and high-quality care, many physicians are just able to do more cases and see more patients than their partners. My suggestion: compensate and applaud them. Everyone will benefit. There's wisdom in the aphorism that "a rising tide lifts all boats."

Communicate, be accountable, and compensate. All are important in fortifying the homeland. All are important in promoting joy and fulfillment in the workplace. All are important in reducing burnout.

We've been spending a lot of time on fortifying the homeland. Let's now finish up and discuss something critically important. Let's finish up in the next chapter by discussing margin.

TEAM TALK

In many clinics and hospital-based settings, the nurses and advanced practice providers are at odds with one another, not working in harmony, or don't necessarily respect administration or their supervising physicians. Quality of care suffers, and the environment promotes burnout.

Healthy communication between providers is important in fortifying the homeland. A positive team communicating with one another is much more successful than an every-man-for-himself mentality. Healthcare and the pressures placed on all providers is too intense to shoulder alone. Team meetings with or without leadership is a wonderful way to build such a successful culture.

Open communication between you and the head nurse, physician, or administration is essential. Unfortunately, many of these leaders are not good leaders and healthy communication with them may depend heavily on you. Remember that being respected flows in both directions, and sometimes needs to be earned before it is granted. Openly disrespecting your boss, either directly or among fellow teammates, is not acceptable—and I have been guilty as charged.

Living in a work environment of "I have no voice, no one is listening to me" is a bad strategy. Resentment and bitterness will eventually spread and be destructive to the homeland. Instead, with humility and well-thought-out words, speak to your boss and share with them your concerns. A unified voice of a number of providers can also be very effective. Even fair compensation can be addressed when a convincing argument is presented in a concise, respectful way.

A Journey Moment

Many physicians find it difficult to keep others accountable. They just put their heads down and keep working harder and harder. In order to help fortify the homeland, list at least three things that you can do to improve accountability, and begin doing them this week. Write down common scenarios and come up with a calm, positive, and well-thought-out strategy to address each one.

1. _____

_____

_____

2. _____

_____

_____

3. _____

_____

_____

CHAPTER 11

FORTIFY THE HOMELAND: MARGIN

A few years ago, I began working in one of our satellite clinics. Initially, I was frustrated at not having access to my usual leaky bladder team, who knew what I liked and how I liked to do things. But I persisted. Gradually, I found that my Mondays at the satellite office were actually enjoyable and so much less stressful than the rest of the week. The difference on Mondays was margin.

At the satellite, I regularly see seven to ten fewer patients than at our main office. I have time to sit and chat with them, I laugh with the nurses, and I don't come unglued when my computer malfunctions. It feels like a different world. I'm no longer sprinting from room to room, and I have a full hour for lunch, which is wonderful. I would never have predicted such a dramatic change in my stress level versus what I consider normal in my regular day-to-day practice.

I know what you're thinking: slowing down and margin is not an option. Trust me, I get it. Read on.

The Answer for Less Burnout

One of the most important ways you can fortify the homeland, especially if you're suffering from burnout or heading in that direction, is to give yourself margin. It's a vital mountaintop decision and one of the most effective and fastest ways to reduce stress as a physician. And yes, it gives you plenty of fist pump opportunities.

In order to give yourself margin as a healthcare provider, you need to reduce your tasks, reduce your exposure, and you need to reduce the grind. **Fewer tasks, less exposure, and less grind are the answers for more joy and less burnout.**

Reduce Your Tasks

The most effective way to reduce tasks is to empower others to do them for you. Train, empower, and give your staff the necessary autonomy. Being the lone ranger is wearing you down and is not sustainable.

Corporatize Decision-Making

I recommend you corporatize the decision-making in your clinic and workplace. Take each functional unit, each nursing station, triage, check-in, etc., and assign a team captain to each.

Any questions regarding tasks or problems are presented to the captain. The captain answers and assists, trains when needed, empowers, and keeps the team accountable. If the captain needs help, he or she approaches the physician or manager during a non-stressful time. Having obtained the solution, the captain teaches the rest of the team. The corporate hierarchy of making decisions is that simple.

Within my clinic, I corporatized decision-making in triage. In addition, I addressed the most common patient questions and requests to have readily available for them. I wrote my protocol, my rules, and importantly, my talk track addressing each one of them. The key: I encouraged triage to make the decision. It was their triage, not mine. I empowered them to be independent, and they appreciated the responsibility.

Bingo. Within two weeks, my tasks from triage decreased by at least 85 percent. It's been wonderful and sustainable. Instead of me giving the same answer to the same question and hitting send to the same person, the triage department make independent decisions and their documented phone messages only need a signature. I sign them with a smile. Fist pump.

Learn to Say No

In addressing my task basket, I needed a healthy change in mindset. I needed to accept that the insatiable appetite of my patients was impossible to satisfy, and therefore I needed healthy boundaries regarding patient behavior. I finally learned that my staff and I had to say no.

It's okay to say no to the patient. It's okay not to oblige their request. We have rules. We have standards. There are two sides to the patient-physician relationship, and patients can always seek care elsewhere if they aren't happy with the boundaries. And don't be fooled by that internal voice tricking you that the referring physician may be upset.

Having boundaries superimposed on attempts to deliver patient-centric excellence has made a significant impact on my staff and myself. For example, patients commonly call for their test results, some hoping to eliminate the need for their follow-up visit. It may be good for them, but it's not good for many providers who are already overwhelmed. "No, I'm sorry, Dr. MacDiarmid does not discuss test results over the phone. The results are important and he believes that they need a face-to-face encounter in order to review." If the patient persists . . . "Discussing test results can be very time consuming, and he is too busy to accommodate these requests." If the patient continues to want the results . . . "We will be happy to send the results to you, but he would need to see you in order to discuss them."

Declaring healthy boundaries and saying no empowers the staff to be more confident and efficient when speaking with patients, reducing the number of tasks generated. It's reduced my frustration and feelings of guilt knowing that it's okay to say no to the patient.

Don't Play the Satisfaction Game

There's no question that the introduction of a Wall Street mentality into the healthcare world now means we have metrics around patient satisfaction. The rationale is that satisfied customers give us repeat business and are a major source of revenue. Patient satisfaction is one of the metrics used by Medicare to reimburse healthcare systems. Encouraged by Obamacare and consultants, driven by money and greed, patient satisfaction and our ability to "make the customer happy" is now a significant source of stress and physician burnout. The intimate patient-physician relationship has been sacrificed for money, a website talking point, a billboard flashing.

Unfortunately, I think many physicians are sensitive when it comes to this feedback and spend too much of their valuable time and energy doing tasks trying to generate an arguably meaningless score in an attempt to make the world satisfied. This month it's a 4.6. Next month, a 4.8. Is this really such an impressive accomplishment to one who has dedicated their life to helping others?

I'm not a player in the world of social media, nor do I pretend that I understand it. But the strategy of assessing our quality of care with a series of likes and dislikes, or now by a key performance indicator used by hospitals, such as patient satisfaction scores, is not a good strategy. In fact, it's a bad strategy.

This satisfaction game is an insult to our profession. It degrades our value as providers. It's no better than the robocall asking you to rate your car salesman, asking for a five-out-of-five score, further propagating the madness.

Stop the madness. Stop checking and worrying about your satisfaction score and online reviews. There is very little to gain from reading them and too much to lose. It's natural for our psyche to be more adversely affected by negative comments than it being lifted up by positivity. Like a parent, your responsibility is not to make your children like you, it's to raise the next generation of loving, honest, and responsible young men and women. For a physician, your job is to use your gifts and talents to help others and to serve with excellence.

So, if your employer or colleague threatens you with negative financial ramifications or recourse for not playing the satisfaction game, remember, you have on your suit of armor.

With humility and shoulders straight, plead your case. Be smart and make reasonable adjustments to accommodate. Carefully seek any constructive criticism. Remind them of your steadfast commitment to delivering patient-centric excellence. But otherwise, politely and professionally tell them no. Tell them to keep the money, that you don't play that game. You are not going to do endless tasks and change how you practice in an attempt to make others happy. **Your personal joy, your self-respect, and your purpose to serve others is not for sale.**

Reduce Your Exposure

Reducing exposure to the ever-increasing and overwhelming patient load is an integral step in the battle to find joy and fight burnout.

Deputize Your Nurse

One day I was sitting in our manager's office and she told me she'd found a replacement for Jill, my nurse and colleague for eight years. Losing Jill was a really big deal. My team's functionality and quality were jeopardized.

"Dr. MacDiarmid, she's young. She has no experience. She just got out of school. She's an accomplished gymnast and coach. But I know you, Dr. MacDiarmid. I know that excellence is so important to you. And I know that you're going to love her. Her name is Jenna." With an affirming and trusting nod, we proceeded to hire her.

Perhaps one of the most effective ways to reduce exposure in your battle against burnout is to deputize your nurse. Jenna has become my shield with my suit of armor.

We have worked to come up with a strategy where she acts as my deputy; shy of any true emergency, nearly all questions for me first go through Jenna. She's my personal triage, my shield. She makes independent decisions. She makes the call. She has my complete trust and protection. Most importantly, when Jenna has a question or concern, she knows when to ask and how to ask. Her words to me are always calming and uplifting.

I'm not asked about adding on a late patient—she decides. Double booking a follow-up? She decides. If triage or the business staff have a question, she triages. There are many times when I observe her making these calls, and I smile in appreciation. Yes, a fist pump moment.

Like any small business, Jenna manages my day-to-day operations. This includes training other staff, following up on tasks given, nipping problems in the bud, and knowing just how to speak to patients. And she is always smiling. So many times I thank Jenna for loving on my patients and helping me deliver excellence.

To my fellow physicians, deputize a trusted person. You need the protection of a shield with your suit of armor. The incoming forces and increasing patient load and demands are overwhelming. The battle to find joy and to fight burnout is too important for you to lose.

Extend Your APPs

The function of physician assistants and nurse practitioners is a fast-growing role, with an increasing number of training programs popping up nationwide. By 2030, it's estimated that the number of advanced practice providers will approach 600,000, greatly outnumbering primary care physicians. Their ever-expanding number is arguably a function of corporatized healthcare.

Initially designed to help extend the care of physicians, their scope of practice and associated independence has greatly increased. And I think in most cases, positively so. There's no question their role is now vital to our patients, to us physicians, and to the function and integrity of the entire healthcare system.

But be careful.

My experience with APPs as they pertain to frustration and burnout is that they can help you or hurt you.

As a perfectionist striving for excellence, there are many times I've bit my lip over sloppy care my patients received from some APPs—to this day I shake my head. Poor care followed by the patient being served back to me like a ping-pong ball just a few weeks later to address the problem, the patient would have been better off just waiting to see me in the first place.

The underlying issue is that in these cases there is too much autonomy and not enough oversight and accountability. Some APPs are not functioning with their intended design and certainly not extending physician excellence. Complaints can be made to partners, but even so, these can be minimized, and the pattern continues, leading to more unacceptable results, frustration, and burnout.

On a much more positive note, when you train, empower, and extend your advanced practice providers to be a functional and multiplying arm of your quality and care, great things can happen. But accountability, along with checks and balances, are a must.

In my quest to give myself margin by reducing my exposure, many of my patients who need follow-up visits within one to three weeks out are seen by my APPs. They extend my care, they extend my treatment pathway, and they do so with a wonderful and comforting smile. Often my patients see Jennaya next, and then follow-up with me a number of weeks afterward. These patients are no longer added to my already full and over-burdened schedule. Less stress. Less burnout. Fist pump.

The Sweet Spot of Scribes

I don't have a scribe, but my gut feeling is to get one. Many claim that once you have a scribe, you won't turn back. If you're burdened by charting and screen time, turn over this endless task to another. Trade hours of documentation with more time spent on your patients. Trade going home late at night with joyful moments with family, friends, and your community. Scribes even help open the door to increasing patient volume and higher revenue.

It is estimated that seeing two extra patients per day will generally cover the cost of your new employee. Scribe agencies exist because it can be difficult to find the right one, and it can be painful when a fully trained and excellent scribe moves on to bigger opportunities, like becoming a nurse, APP, or other.

I think there's a sweet spot when using scribes, especially for those who are battling with or tending toward burnout. While it's tempting to significantly increase your volume with a scribe's help, more patients mean more tasks, more burden, and more responsibility. For me, significantly more is not my sweet spot.

And the quality of your documentation may be jeopardized when entered primarily by others. With the quality of notes already threatened by templates, cutting and pasting, and text added to satisfy billing requirements, I encourage you to not let your scribed notes deteriorate further. They may be able to document the interaction, but they may not be able to capture your thoughts, which may just be the most valuable part of the note.

The Scribe Hybrid

My solution is to train a medical provider with typing skills to function as my clinical scribe extender. I guess you could say a Jenna hybrid. A medical assistant or nurse who can type, dictate, help answer tasks, and even take histories. One who can help with patient care as well as education. I would be willing to pay more, allowing me to find a higher skilled person and one who stays longer.

Similar to working with a junior resident, the two of us would share the daily clinical and clerical duties, varying our approach with each patient. This would give me a modest increase in volume, more quality time with patients, less burdensome clerical duties, and coming home sooner, smiling, with a few extra dollars in my pocket. Yes, that's the sweet spot.

Dictate

Many burnout experts recommend for physicians to become computer super-users to improve their efficiency and to reduce frustration. Not being one places me at a disadvantage. There's no question that the more you develop your ability to navigate and troubleshoot, you are more proficient and less likely to decompensate when the computer malfunctions.

On a bad day, computer issues can be a tremendous source of stress. Redundant functionality, too many boxes to open and click, invalid passwords—the list goes on. And if your IT support has been outsourced overseas to save a few bucks, stop the madness! You're going to blow a gasket. Have IT support onsite or immediately available.

I think there's nothing better than dictating a comprehensive note. This is the closest we can come to capturing thought. State-of-the-art voice recognition software now provides reasonable access to quality, completeness, and speed. Too often quality is sacrificed when typing, because even the speedsters cut corners.

Templates are also time savers, but again, be careful. I use them to document my lengthy surgical consent discussions, but otherwise I don't like them. I find them too robotic and believe they threaten the art of medicine and important details of the patient encounter.

While it's not in my top ten issues, many physicians should be ashamed of themselves when it comes to their cut-and-paste and template charting. Seriously, the quality of the history of present illness and discussion sections in many notes I receive from others is just awful. I think to some degree it's a part of physicians commoditizing patients, and for others it's a sign of burnout. I encourage all of us to try to do better.

Limit Care over the Phone

My partner was on the phone with a patient, and as the minutes went by, he repeated the same information over and over again. More minutes went by, and now the phone was turned over from the spouse to the actual patient. He repeated the information for a third time. Finally, he was able to hang up after a lengthy conversation. Wow, this was so giving on his part, but so taking on the part of the patient and his spouse.

Of course it's important to speak to patients over the phone, but I recommend that you limit phone calls as much as possible, unless it's a telehealth visit. In my experience, the calls tend to ramble on, they self-generate unrelated issues, and quality of care sometimes deteriorates. The patient is often left with questions and is less satisfied. If you don't believe me, ask one of your nurses who regularly experiences these calls. My general policy not to give care over the phone has been a good one.

In my opinion, MyChart is a disaster for many employed physicians forced to use it by their corporatized system. I'm thankful that I don't have to answer endless patient emails and requests generated by them reading their chart. The back and forth, the inefficiencies, the tail absolutely wagging the dog. It might be good for patient satisfaction, but what about me?

And I'll throw in a word of caution to my fellow surgeons who get patients to consent to surgery over the phone. There's nothing safer and better than a face-to-face encounter for the preoperative consent. Remember, if a lawsuit occurs, you need everything in your favor and to keep exposure limited. You are about to embark on a surgical journey often associated with pain, suffering, and uncertainty: have the patient make the decision face-to-face.

On Call

I sometimes joke that next to your latest EMR update going live, the two most painful words in medicine are *on call*. For many specialists, it's a tremendous source of stress. I think that many doctors, already fatigued and discouraged by their day jobs, don't have the emotional reserve to easily handle it. I've heard physicians cite that no longer wanting to be on call was their primary reason for early retirement.

A couple of thoughts on how to get through being on call. First, when on call, survival is your number one priority. **I recommend a survival mentality for the days you're on call if you find them stressful.** At the beginning of each on-call period, I have four goals: survival, providing excellence, gratitude, and trying to smile with each and every patient. My goals are rehearsed during call mornings as I'm putting on my suit of armor. Attempts to maximize work relative value units and income, or to do other projects while on call, is not a good strategy.

I also recommend reducing your exposure. There's no question that if you're struggling with physician burnout that decreasing your exposure while on call can go a long way in fortifying the homeland. Armed with a survival mentality, I urge you to take actionable steps in order to give yourself necessary margin.

Remember your goals. And when successful, with or without sleep, when your call is over, don't forget the fist pump. Mission accomplished.

On-Call Margin-Building Steps:

Reduce your template. When I reduced my office template by 50 percent during call days, it made such a difference. It gave me the necessary margin to absorb work-ins and to accommodate urgent hospital consults. My neck muscles relaxed. I had less stress and anxiety. Looking back, a full patient load while being on call was just not worth it.

Cancel and reschedule. Too often, I see partners on call leaving clinic and rushing off to address an urgent consult. Emergencies arise at a moment's notice. Then they return to a waiting room full of frustrated or angry patients who have been waiting hours for their appointment. And the doctor is frazzled and stressed, eyes crying out for help, and the flames of burnout blazing.

My policy differs. Recognizing the inconvenience to patients, I decided a few years ago to change my practice and decided to prioritize my health and stress level over others. Being Superman and trying to accommodate everyone possible was just not worth it.

So, in such circumstances, I cancel and reschedule clinic when I need to leave urgently. I don't mind if those cancelled are double-booked to see me the following day, or soon thereafter. My policy gives me margin and frees my mind so that I can now be fully engaged in attending to the emergency situation. It works and it's calming. Liberate yourselves and your waiting room; you have the power.

Patients who have acute needs or select personal circumstances who can't wait until the next day—with their permission—should sit and wait for my return. Or better still, a partner or nurse practitioner agrees to step in, which provides a wonderful rescue for the patient.

Utilize your APPs. Our APPs are the first line of defense in evaluating and treating same-day work-ins, especially established patients. At least for specialists, patient expectations have made many call days feel like a walk-in clinic, with very few cases being urgent or semi-urgent. Patients want service and they want it now. APPs help accommodate this new world of commoditized care.

Just call me Canadian. I have no idea why physicians in the U.S. have allowed patients to call us in the middle of the night to tell us their testicles have been sore for months, or that their prescription needs renewal. In my home country of Canada, physicians are on call to the emergency department, and they are not called directly by patients. There's no question that the public has taken advantage of this luxury with more of them calling us 24-7.

The studies on sleep clearly demonstrate that the quality of sleep directly correlates with daily function and the overall health and well-being of an individual.

Physicians on call need their sleep. It's our duty to be highly functional when needed for an emergency. Remember, it's safety first. We cannot continue to sacrifice ourselves and, potentially, quality of care in our failing attempts to make everyone happy and satisfied. Let me provide you with two suggestions in order to avoid these calls.

First, don't personally answer patient calls after hours. Instead, use an independent call service, or more commonly, use your APPs or nurses to triage. If needed, compensate them for doing so. When our group adopted this, it made a big difference to our physicians' health and sanity. The additional sleep was wonderful.

Second, I like what a urology group in Florida has done regarding this matter. Their patients are proactively educated regarding office policies, including the handling of after-hour calls. Setting appropriate expectations is important.

So, if a patient calls in the middle of the night, the message reminds them that the office is closed and that any perceived urgencies should be addressed in the emergency room. Otherwise, they should call back during open hours. Importantly, patients who have had surgery or a procedure in the last thirty days are instructed to stay on the line to speak to someone.

Pay for call. Fortunately, more and more hospitals are now compensating physicians for being on call. I must say, what a blessing. There's no question that receiving financial reward for your extra effort positively impacts one's psyche. I believe it also helps open the doors of trust and appreciation, both important to the physician-hospital relationship.

I recommend that you negotiate a win-win agreement with your hospital if you're not already getting compensated. For instance, when we started staffing a satellite hospital for our healthcare system, they agreed to compensate us for on call, and everyone benefitted. I believe that pay-for-call helps fortify the homeland and fights physician burnout.

Write the check. One of the best things I did to minimize my exposure in my battle against burnout was paying my younger partners to take some of my call days, specifically weekends. With us already being reimbursed by the hospital, I paid handsomely in addition to what they were paying, and it really has been a win-win.

As a result, I no longer work weekends and my total call burden has lessened by nearly 50 percent. The strategy has been very beneficial. As I write the check, never with a second thought and always with gratitude, I look up. Fist pump.

Reduce the Grind

We've covered two ways to give yourself margin—reduce the tasks and reduce exposure. The third way to give yourself margin and fortify your homeland is you're going to have to reduce the grind. Our profession must start thinking differently about how we practice, but more importantly, how we protect and nurture ourselves. This is serious business.

Be Like Doug

During my recent physical, my primary care physician told me that things at his practice were going pretty well with him and his partners, and specifically when it came to physician joy and burnout. Quite frankly I was a bit surprised and curious, so I enquired further.

He told me that compensation had recently improved because they'd joined an accountable care organization, in addition to negotiating some better contracts. Certainly Doug had figured a few things out and still enjoyed looking after patients as their primary care provider.

And then he stopped. "Oh, Scott. But I forgot to tell you that we're now only working four days a week. There's no way I could do this job Monday through Friday. It's much too stressful! I'd burn out."

Doug, a model physician who loves his patients, wisely realized that he needs regular time off in order for him to get recharged and be joyful.

Many physicians need to do the same and reduce the grind by shortening their work week. Take three days to recover. Three days to live on their mountaintop with family, friends, community, and nurture their personal health. Three days to help balance the work week.

I believe that most physicians could make 90 percent of their income working four days a week by being efficient and strategic. Be like Doug: work four days a week, and give yourself the necessary margin by reducing the grind.

See Fewer People

As a once high producer in my group, I prided myself in my ability to efficiently and effectively see a large number of patients. In many cases, they had complicated problems. I limited the chit-chat, stayed totally on task, and with my stride lengthened, my clinic really moved.

But after years of such service, I found myself fatigued, more edgy, and more impatient. I had less reserve to absorb the speed bumps. I started regularly counting the number of patients left on my schedule and wishing the day was over.

I finally decided to reduce my template and see fewer patients. My trusted team reorganized new and return visits to improve efficiency, and we reduced the number of afternoon slots, guaranteeing me a four o'clock departure. For others, it may be better to work to day's end, but reduce the number of patients seen per hour.

I love leaving early to go off to the gym and enjoy an evening with my family. My nurses also appreciate that hour at the end of the day to catch up with the seemingly never-ending nursing duties. I can see their fist pumps now.

Provide Exit Strategies

I think it's important for our profession to start thinking differently about how we practice. How we grind it out to the end and push ourselves until we get ill or retire. For many, it's not a good strategy.

We need to start providing exit strategies, not only for those soon-to-retire, but for the many burning out who are not going to make it the length of their working life and are suffering and miserable. I have a couple of suggestions.

If surgery is too stressful, become an office-based physician. Speak to your partners, change your compensation model, and stop doing surgery or the types of cases that are stressing you. Work as a team and accommodate. We all have tremendous value and need the caring and understanding of one another.

For others, a nice win-win formula is to job share. Two physicians providing great care as one practice, both working half time can be life-giving to many.

But beware: usually for others to agree to exiting strategies, you likely will be expected to shoulder your fair share of the negatives, including being on call, and there will be financial ramifications associated. Otherwise, slowing down at the perceived expense of others is not going to be successful. You cannot expect to have your cake and eat it too.

You Don't Need a Range Rover

So far, my advice in this section has been to slow down, work four days a week, and reduce your template. Exit strategies. I know what you're thinking: How can I afford to do this? But let me address your concerns.

Yes, you will likely need to sacrifice a higher income in order to slow down and to give yourself margin. Some might be masters of efficiency and can likely do so and remain nearly budget neutral.

But if you're burning out, please don't put a price tag on your personal health and joy. Don't put a price tag on your relationships with family, friends, and your community. Listen, you don't need a Range Rover. Trade in your Range Rover and standard of living for a little bit less. Trade it for living on your mountaintop and finishing strong.

And as my friend David commonly says, "Scott, when are you going to realize that the sweet spot in medicine is when an overperformer like yourself learns to underperform?" It's sad but it's true. Many of us are killing ourselves overperforming and too many are burning out trying to do so.

Go home and build your legacy at home. Go home and watch your daughter play volleyball. Go home and walk your dog with your beautiful wife. Go home and be grateful that you put in another day and accomplished your mission of serving others. Fist pump.

You see, ladies and gentlemen, your family, friends, community, and your health are all critical to fuel your journey to your mountaintop. Without them, you simply cannot reach the summit.

TEAM TALK

Nurses and APPs need margin in order to fortify the homeland. Reducing your tasks, exposure, and the grind are important strategies, enabling you to fight burnout and to experience joy when caring for patients. Many margin builders overlap with those already discussed in this chapter, but let me make a few additional comments.

Corporatizing decision-making within each functional unit is a successful strategy. Problem-solving and answering tasks without needing to speak with supervisors or physicians saves time and improves efficiency. It also promotes personal growth and satisfaction. Such a decision-making process within a hospital setting will likely need additional approval from others. But I encourage you to push through any temporary roadblocks, since the mission is important.

Ask your physician or supervisor for their talk tracks and protocols for how they want common circumstances handled at a nursing or APP level. Let the hierarchy know that you want to make independent decisions within the guard-rails of the system and in doing so everyone will benefit. If needed, write down your own ideas and present them to the appropriate person for endorsement.

Fill up a binder with helpful notes, pre-authorization success stories, clinical pathways, troubleshooting tips, etc., and make them as specific as possible. My two nurses have binders—I refer to them as their "bibles of excellence." Make additions and modify your notes as necessary and share them with colleagues. Don't be afraid to make suggestions on how to improve care and efficiency. Medicine is a team sport, and your perspective is priceless.

Reducing tasks by learning to say no is vital for nurses and APPs. Be kind, precise, but to the point when speaking with patients. Identifying with a patient's needs is important, especially when they are stressed or upset, but having boundaries with a guiding star of delivering excellence will protect you and save precious time and emotional energy.

All providers who are computer super-users are advantaged and less suscep-tible to being bogged down and stressed by electronic medical records. But even if you are a proficient typist, don't hesitate to dictate. Any perceived cost associated with transcription will be more than justified by your ability to see a few more patients. And remember that scribes can also help advanced practice providers be more efficient.

Reducing the grind by working fewer and perhaps longer days or by working part time is a lifeline for many. The extra days off provide time needed for rest and renewal.

Don't be afraid to change nursing or APP jobs if things are stale, stressful, or no longer rewarding. A fresh challenge or new environment will invigorate many. Transitioning from hospital to office-based care can eliminate many stressors and improve working hours. Don't feel guilty for choosing a less demanding setting or career—your health and well-being is much more precious.

Diversifying your nursing career by splitting clinical care with perhaps educational, academic, or administrative duties has been demonstrated to successfully reduce stress. Many nurses have exit strategies, including becoming an APP, a certified registered nurse anesthetist, a full-time administrator, a pharmaceutical sales representative, and many more. Nurses have so many wonderful talents to share with others.

A Journey Moment

It's time that you begin providing yourself some margin so you can be less stressed and happier. Carefully read this chapter again. Underline or mark all margin builders that you can implement. Make a list. Come up with a strategy and get started. Fist pump.

1. _____
2. _____
3. _____
4. _____
5. _____
6. _____
7. _____

CHAPTER 12

BECOME A BETTER FIGHTER BY BEING MORE EFFICIENT

There is no question that many physicians are overwhelmed by the clerical demands and inefficiencies associated with treating patients in the new world of healthcare. In an attempt to see the same number of patients, providers are mentally exhausted, and their days significantly lengthened in order to accommodate the new ways in which we have to process all the paperwork.

We have to come in early to prime the day's charts, and then we have to stay late to dictate the patient visits and answer messages. Unfortunately, many of us take work home to complete during evenings and weekends. And Monday morning, the never-ending cycle starts all over again.

And for what? Year after year there is less compensation, more stress and regulations, more tasks to complete, and more burnout. We are like hamsters on a wheel, a cog in the healthcare system. An unfortunate end for some of the most gifted, hard-working, and smartest individuals.

Learn to be Efficient

Some physicians are much more able to navigate the system in spite of its demands. They adapt, they adjust, they get things done efficiently while still maintaining quality. I guess you could say that in the fight against burnout, they've learned to become better fighters by being more efficient.

Let me share with you a number of combat techniques that could make you more efficient in navigating your day's work. Some methods and mindsets might equip you to fight better. We're all different. We all have our own style and work circumstances. But I think we can all learn from one another, and even small adjustments at work for some could make a big difference.

Efficiency Begins with a Mindset

First and foremost, efficient behavior begins with a mindset that you are no longer going to sacrifice your life working long hours to accommodate the system. Those days are over.

You're a doctor, not a clerical worker. It's time to have boundaries and to say no.

Define your work hours and design a system to suit. Make adjustments, use fortifying-the-homeland techniques, and learn to become more efficient. Small efficiencies that maintain quality when multiplied are time-saving and life-giving. Let's discuss.

Become Algorithmic

An algorithm is a step-by-step procedure for solving a logical and mathematical problem or accomplishing some end. A recipe is a good example, because step by step it directs you on what has to be done. I think some physicians are more wired than others to be algorithmic, but the skill can be learned.

Dating back to my residency, including time spent at Duke and overseas, I was trained to be algorithmic when treating patients. And in my earlier days as an emergency room physician, algorithms were the norm.

To this day, I place most of my patients on a step-by-step treatment pathway, consciously or subconsciously. It directs and organizes my care, it's efficient, and it drives excellence. And there's no question there's less stress when you have a defined plan of action for each patient, in spite of the complexity. The step-by-step plan keeps you focused, and this is key to not getting derailed.

When necessary, spend more time dissecting the patient's initial complaints since it will save you time in the long run. Define and dictate a diagnostic and treatment pathway or multiple ones, paths that occur simultaneously or perhaps sequentially.

For example, I may have a patient who complains of recurrent urinary tract infections, urinary incontinence, and vague back pain. The patient has their own description of their problems, but it is up to me to organize each problem into a focused diagnostic and treatment plan. I control the conversation, focus on and dissect each complaint, and then define my algorithm for each.

On the front end, I recommend a few extra questions if needed, being as specific as possible for each problem. I liberally order clinically important diagnostic tests. Remember, a step-by-step process for each patient complaint will focus you and help deliver excellence. And it's on the front end that the algorithm is best defined and dictated.

Resist the temptation of shotgun empiric therapy medicine. Resist writing a prescription for a bunch of poorly defined symptoms, hoping that you can just move on to the next patient. Failure rates are high. Excellent care is lacking. The patient may return frustrated and often with the same list of problems, bogging you down even more. They may also have the sense that you never listened to them in the first place.

And if you're relying on your poorly documented cut and pasted templated medical records, your return visit can be much more time-consuming and challenging. Every patient starts feeling like a new patient. You have nothing valuable in your notes. It's no wonder your day is falling apart; it's no wonder your clinic is inefficient.

In contrast, when patients are on a treatment path, follow-up visits are much more organized and fulfilling. It's clear where the patient is situated in their therapeutic pathway, which is quickly summarized to them like a story during each visit. Doctor and patient are all on the same page, all on the same pathway, and quality goes up and stress goes down.

The same step-by-step algorithm documented in the medical record also makes trouble-shooting and patient questions and tasks from staff much easier to navigate. A quick look at where the patient is in their pathway and you'll know exactly how to respond.

Many patients reach their treatment goal somewhere along the pathway, while others choose to abandon the journey. Of course, some reach the end the algorithm without success and unfortunately have no other treatment options available. This is reality.

Stop throwing the dart and become algorithmic. It's efficient. It drives excellence. It's fulfilling. Algorithms don't turn patients into numbers. Paradoxically, it simplifies the complex data of medicine, and allows you more time and brain space to connect with the human before you. A mathematical approach to medicine will increase joy and reduce burnout.

Know When to Punt and Move On

Even with a well-documented treatment path, you can still get bogged down by challenging or complex patients. It's also easy to get overwhelmed by patient demands and unhappiness, a complication, or a lengthy run when there are no easy patient visits in your day.

Already an hour behind, spending forty minutes with the next patient is not only fatiguing and stressful, but I believe when chronic, promotes burnout. One effective strategy to counteract this is knowing when to punt and move on to the next patient.

Obviously, you can't solve or address all problems during a single sitting, and don't be afraid to be transparent with your patient about this fact. In my experience, patients are satisfied as long as they know the issue will be dealt with eventually. Addressing erectile dysfunction during the same visit as an elevated PSA is not efficient.

Avoid a complete patient assessment with review of their extensive medical records, a complete clinical evaluation, and discussion of all treatment options during one encounter. You cannot understand years of problems and come up with and communicate instant cures in minutes. Be clear about expectations, and steadily march forward one step at a time. Overly ambitious expectations will suffocate your clinic. And over time, these lengthy visits will weaken even the best of fighters.

Punt complicated therapeutic and extensive surgical discussions to the next visit, especially when a trial of conservative therapy or another test is needed. I promise you, you'll be asked to repeat the same discussion during the follow-up visit.

Avoid operating on the first date; it's a bad strategy. Take your time, punt, bring the patient back for a final surgery discussion. Building relationships and setting expectations is important before offering a scalpel.

Don't be tempted to schedule an operation on day one by the "I just want it fixed now" patient. He or she will often be the most disappointed when they don't reach their treatment goal with surgery. Your nonsurgical recommendations and their rush to operate will have never happened. You'll be blamed. It will be your fault. The patient will not share any of the responsibility.

There's wisdom in punting. Punting reduces stress, and wear and tear. One punt can send you home thirty minutes early with less fatigue and frustration. There's no question that knowing when to punt makes you a better fighter.

Control the Conversation

Unfortunately, physicians are under increasing pressure to see more and more patients and have less and less time for each. Less time threatens quality of care, but also takes away from us getting to know our patients, personal things that promote joy and trust in the patient-physician relationship. Things that nourish us as physicians.

Having said that, I've elected to spend most of my minutes staying on task, concentrating on the medical problem. I try to use close-ended questions that can be sensibly answered with either a yes or no, with a provided choice, or with a specific short response. Even with that, commonly the responses are tangential and don't even come close to answering the question. I think that in my case, many patients are not used to discussing their bladders and have difficulty describing the problem. Sometimes this proves frustrating, but I persist.

I try to direct and control the conversation in a kind, empathetic, and conversational manner.

For good or bad, I do interrupt, and my residents tease me that I'm the master of limiting patient ramble and unnecessary discussion. Spending time on vague and unrelated complaints with an anxious patient is not beneficial for either of us. Bottom line: I need the facts and I will not sacrifice quality.

Controlling the conversation is efficient, saves time, and provides a quality outcome. Remember that two minutes of extra chit-chat per patient, times thirty patients a day equates to having enough time to spend with all of your patients and still leave the office with positive attitude, and enough time for a workout at the end of the day. Yes, two minutes of being more efficient will make you a better fighter.

But unfortunately, there's a price to the way I practice. I think I would have more joy and fulfillment if I sat and chatted more with my patients. It's a tough balance and likely varying your approach according to the individual patient and the day's circumstances is preferred.

And to those physicians who can take forty-five minutes to evaluate and to get to know a new patient, cheers to you! But unfortunately, most surgeons and specialists simply don't have this luxury.

Develop a Team Approach

Close proximity to my nursing team provides me the necessary environment to be maximumly efficient. With my team only feet apart at our workstations, the three "cooks" in our "kitchen" speak back and forth, and the team functions beautifully.

The three of us share clinic duties, schedule follow-ups, send electronic prescriptions, locate referral notes—the menu is long. Who does what depends on patient volume, and on minute-by-minute circumstances. For me to spend a few extra minutes on clerical duties while a nurse sits idle is inefficient, especially when two more patients are waiting in rooms. The team goal is: be efficient, be excellent, and get the head chef out the door by four o'clock.

Communication is key. It fosters a team atmosphere and empowers excellence. I call out orders and instructions to my nurses, and with their verbal confirmation, I finish my dictation and I'm off to see the next patient.

In contrast, I see excellent partners getting bogged down, shouldering too many of their tasks and duties, while several yards away their nurses sit idling. This is not an efficient strategy while there are patients waiting, and no one is happy.

Most days our team approach provides me with multiple brief opportunities to address emails and other tasks that always accumulate. Get rid of these accumulators as you work throughout the day.

It's time to become a better fighter and to be more efficient. Become algorithmic. Know when to punt. Control the conversation. Be cooks in a kitchen with a team approach. These are all combat techniques that can make you a better fighter. A better fighter who goes home on time with tasks completed.

Fist pump.

TEAM TALK

Nurses and APPs can identify with the never-ending clerical needs, longer hours, and working harder to meet the demands of commoditized healthcare. Too many come in early and go home late, and one wonders if it's sustainable. Being a hamster on the wheel running faster and faster is overwhelming and exhausting.

All providers can learn to be better fighters and more efficient, enabling them to deliver excellent care while maintaining personal quality of life. Success begins with the mindset that you are willing to work hard, but not sacrifice your joy and health to accommodate the system.

Nurses are commonly bombarded with of list of symptoms and patient complaints when delivering patient care and triaging phone calls. Being algorithmic by asking a few additional questions and placing the patient on a diagnostic or treatment pathway keeps you focused, is less stressful, and provides excellence.

Knowing when to punt is important, especially when you are stressed and overwhelmed. In the midst of the day's chaos, punt the patient or family member on the phone who otherwise would talk forever. Having boundaries and letting them know that you will call them later can satisfy many. Controlling the conversation and blending it with empathy and respect saves time and is effective.

Being in close proximity to your supervising physician and other providers is a good team strategy. All cooks in the kitchen benefit when the day's menu and its endless tasks are shared. Good communication promotes a team atmosphere and delivers great care.

Think of all the fist pumps when you learn to fight better.

A Journey Moment

Do you regularly come in early, go home late, or take work home with you during nights and weekends?

_____

_____

_____

_____

_____

_____

If so, do you think that it's negatively impacting you or your family?

If yes, is it time for a new mindset? Is it time to draw a line in the sand and say no?

Can you think of ways of becoming more efficient and being a better fighter? If yes, write down three and implement them. And don't forget the fist pumps.

1. _____

2. _____

3. _____

Chapter 13

Rethinking the Battle

There seems to be a disconnect between having such a joyful and fulfilling career as a physician and burning out on it. Let me explain.

You could argue that the profession of medicine, like no other, is an amazing opportunity to be happy and satisfied. Just think about it: on a daily basis, we use our gifts and talents to help others. We sacrifice for the health and well-being of our communities. For so many, it's our calling.

I think our calling is why we're willing to give so much of our lives to our work. Just think of the training, the family time missed, holidays on call, the daily burdens and stress. Fulfilling one's calling brings joy, meaning, and purpose. And purpose justifies the hardships.

So, why are so many of us not joyful? Recognizing that most physicians are pretty tough individuals who went through intense training, why are the difficulties of practicing medicine arguably no longer worth it, or wearing us down?

Do We Have the Right Battle Strategy?

Of course the answer is complex, multifactorial, and reasons differ among individuals. Answers might be that our profession became devalued, providers are no longer respected, death by a thousand cuts, etc.

But I believe there's a deeper problem. For many, the problem is not having the right battle strategy. Many physicians rely on others for their joy and fulfillment—and this is not wise or effective. It's a battle strategy that we can't win.

We might have approached the position saying, "Yes we'll help, yes we'll sacrifice, but there are conditions to the social contract." We need others to be thankful and respectful. We need to be well compensated. We need electronic medical records to function adequately.

Whether placing such conditions is right or wrong is debatable, but I'm here to point out that perhaps there's a flaw in our thinking as it pertains to our rules of engagement. We're relying on third-party payers, patients, hospitals, and even the government to change their behavior in order for us to be fulfilled and to battle burnout.

That means we're depending on others to bring the solution to our problem. And, ladies and gentlemen, we need to be realistic. The negative forces that are stealing our joy and promoting physician burnout unfortunately are likely to continue, and in many cases will only worsen.

A better battle strategy is to accept the cards that we've been dealt. To accept the circumstances we find ourselves in. In doing so, we can then define our own mountaintop and make decisions that align ourselves with our upward ascent and stop doing things that drag us down into the valley.

I believe that taking such responsibility is a better battle strategy for ourselves, for our friends and family, and for our patients and community. At first glance, this might seem daunting, but it's actually quite liberating, because it gives us control over our own destiny. It gives us control over living our purpose of serving others and over our ability to finish strong.

When I finally changed my battle strategy to focus on myself and on my upward climb to the summit and stopped dwelling on the external forces that were tearing me down, it truly was a turning point in my life in finding joy as a practicing clinician. **Taking personal responsibility has made me a much better climber.**

Have We Identified the Right Battlefield?

I had a cartoon: picture a hulk of a man—a real warrior—fiercely carving a path through a dense forest with an enormous machete. On a mission to construct a path to the other side, he wielded his weapon faster and faster. With each blow, almost frantic, one great tree after another fell with a thunderous crash.

Two other places of observation were depicted. The aerial view was revealing. It showed that the path the man was making had no end. The forest went on forever. A man on a mission, he was never going to reach his destination. And being in the midst of dense timberland, he was unaware of that. As time lengthened, he swung harder, he swung faster. He was probably getting fatigued.

On a tall ladder, a second man stood at the path's beginning. Peering over the trees, it gave him perspective. His binoculars exaggerated in size, his cartoon eyes vividly apparent, he uttered, "Wrong forest."

Well, that leads us to another reason why physicians answering their calling may still not be joyful.

In rethinking the battle against burnout, I started wondering if physicians have identified the right battlefield. Or are we swinging our machetes harder and faster, but in the wrong forest? And some of us are getting fatigued.

Perhaps we've given too much of our lives and place too much of our lives purpose on the practice of medicine, making our job our battlefield. And that might not be the best strategy. The more I think about it, for many it's an unwise strategy because it might be a battle that we cannot win.

Many physicians live their lives out of balance. Robotically, we're programmed to do so during training, when the demands and hours of the job are endless. We work, we work, and we work, often without adequate sleep.

For many, medicine is a way of life and not just an occupation. The office and hospital become our life. All of our friends are at work, and we often just go home to sleep and to get ready for the next day. Maybe it's not possible to feel fulfilled in life primarily through one's job, as opposed to seeking fulfillment through multiple life domains, like family, friends, physical and mental/spiritual health, and community.

Experts claim that we need to be well-grounded in the majority of these domains in order to be fulfilled. Physicians, so overwhelmed with work, lack depth in a number of the other domains. In many cases, we sacrifice them for work. But what happens to our joy and fulfillment when our job lets us down—what else do we have if we haven't built anything else in our lives?

To live a mountaintop life we must include all five domains. We must learn to seek fulfillment in all aspects of life, and we must prioritize differently at times in order to do so. We must make mountaintop decisions in each of them, aligning ourselves with our summit, and stop doing things that pull us down into the valley.

Perhaps then we'll find meaning in life. When tribulations occur in one or more of the domains, including those associated with the practice of medicine, it might be tolerable and worth enduring when you look at your entire life's picture.

So I think it's prudent for us to ask, "Are we in the wrong forest? Are we swinging our machetes harder and faster, but with no victory in sight?" I don't know about you, but with every decade passing, my attempt to swing that machete is becoming more and more tiring.

Instead, some of us need a tall ladder and some oversized binoculars that provide us with an aerial view of a much healthier and even nobler perspective. An aerial view of the right battlefield.

Are We Wired for the Battle?

Clinical psychologists commonly speak about the Big 5 personality traits, describing what they believe are the five basic dimensions of personality. The traits comprise different degrees of extroversion, conscientiousness, agreeableness, neuroticism, and openness.

Extroverts enjoy interacting with people and are perceived as being full of energy. They're outgoing, they're expressive, they're the louder ones in the group.

Second only to IQ, conscientiousness is the highest predictor for success in academics and many professions, such as law and medicine. Those high in conscientiousness are hardworking, believe that structure and rules are important, they have integrity, and they drive excellence.

Those high in agreeableness are compassionate and want to help and to serve. Placing others before themselves is common.

Those high in neuroticism are more negatively impacted with worry and anxiety when given the same levels of stress as another person.

People ranked high in openness are creative, think outside of the box— they're the musicians, the inventors, and the entrepreneurs.

I wondered if there are personality traits that equip you well to being a physician, or more importantly, predispose an individual to burn out? I've concluded that the answer is yes.

If you're going to go to war to fight burnout and find joy, you should know if your personality is wired for the battle. Because if you are not, without some rewiring, you might have a tough go of it.

Let me use myself as an example. I'm high in extroversion, conscientiousness, and agreeableness, low in neuroticism, and at best, moderate in openness.

As an extrovert, practicing medicine and being a surgeon is a great job for me since I interact with so many on a daily basis.

Being high in conscientiousness, I now realize that in almost everything I do, I try to deliver excellence. I'm sure that's why I became a subspecialist, where excellence is easier to attain. This also might explain why I'm on a mission to arm myself with as much knowledge and skill as possible to help and encourage others to find joy in the workplace. The way I see the complexity of this subject is that I'm just getting started.

Like most physicians, being high in agreeableness is in my genetic code to serve and to help others. No matter the struggles, I know the three-quarters-length white lab coat was made for me.

But importantly, my wiring shines the light on why I struggle with burnout.

129

Mediocrity, the same person asking me the same question, the dumbing down of the American healthcare system, all play havoc with my conscientiousness. On a bad day it can drive me crazy.

Programmed to be a doer, for years my conscientiousness meant that I attempted to solve problems, including emotional ones, by doing *more*. And guess what? In many cases it didn't work.

The profession of medicine is filled with highly conscientious individuals. The problem is that conscientious people are generally not good in adapting to changing environments, they just keep doing what they know. So, is it any wonder that physicians have had a hard time adapting to the new world of healthcare?

My agreeableness explains why I get hurt or easily angered by an ungrateful patient; their words pierce a knife into me. People high in agreeableness are often taken advantage of by those who are not, and as a result are prone to feeling resentful.

If you think about it, the personality traits that help equip us to be good physicians simultaneously expose us to burnout. This is especially so when we're unaware of our wiring and don't know how to manage ourselves effectively. Let me give you three thoughts to consider.

First, your personality is the prism through which you see and process the world. It explains to some degree why you react or don't react. It influences your value structure and dictates how you define your mountaintop and find meaning.

Knowledge of your personality or wiring better equips you to make mountaintop decisions that nourish your personality and avoid the actions and decisions that starve you and pull you down into the valley of burnout.

Second, experts recommend that you develop some attributes on the opposite end of each of the five personality traits spectrum. You cannot change your basic personality, but you can rewire yourself to some degree. Such rewiring will help protect you, will make you more adaptable, and it's an effective way to mature and become wiser.

So, an agreeable person who learns to be more disagreeable when appropriate is more apt to stand up for themselves and therefore limit the amount of resentment they feel. When an overly conscientious person learns to accept imperfections, he or she often finds themselves happier. Just chilling a bit makes them less judgmental and frustrated by lower performers. Extroverts who learn that they don't need to tell the world every time they are frustrated or angry will benefit themselves and others. When a neurotic person learns to be positive and realizes that there is a brighter side to most circumstances, their stress will lessen.

Third, having knowledge of, acceptance of, and nourishing the differences in the personality traits of fellow physicians can be an actionable step forward for healthier group dynamics and fortifying the homeland. Partners that you may regularly knock heads with are often not bad folks, they are just wired and see the world differently.

Here are some basic group dynamic suggestions: listen more to the agreeable who perceive themselves as being silenced or minimized; acknowledge and reward the conscientious one, who may be frustrated as an over-producer; be open to the ideas of the rare creative, they may change the world.

Recognize the wiring of everyone in the group. Listen, acknowledge, and be open. All of these efforts could go a long way in fortifying the homeland and reducing burnout. All could go a long way in making the group more successful, more joyful, and yes, more profitable.

TEAM TALK

It's important for nurses and APPs to rethink the battle, especially as it relates to having the right battle strategy, identifying the right battlefield, and assessing whether they are wired for the task in hand.

Nurses who wait for patients and their families to be kind and respectful in order to feel fulfilled may be disappointed and miss out on their calling to joyfully serve others.

The manager of one of our clinics recently gave great advice to the staff and providers about work/life balance. She reminded them that this is a job and not your life. She emphasized that meaning and joy extend far beyond the workplace.

Understanding your personality as it pertains to the five personality traits and how it relates to caring for patients is important for all providers. And by recognizing and developing the areas of your personality on the other side of the spectrum that do not come naturally, you will be more successful in interacting with patients and colleagues.

A JOURNEY MOMENT

Do you have the right battle strategy? Are you relying on conditions or others to change in order for you to be joyful and fulfilled? If yes, write down one external force that regularly wears you down that you now accept. Consider repeating this exercise weekly.

_____

_____

_____

_____

_____

Have you identified the right battlefield? Have you placed too much emphasis on practicing medicine at the expense of other life domains? If yes, identify one thing that you will start doing in another domain that will nourish you or those around you.

_____

_____

_____

_____

_____

FIST PUMPS

Are you wired for the battle? And do you need some rewiring in order to battle burnout and to find joy? If yes, identify the personality trait that needs rewiring and strategize how you will make some changes.

_____

_____

_____

_____

_____

_____

_____

Part 3: Effectively Managing the Greed Virus

By identifying the healthcare crisis and learning successful battle strategies in parts 1 and 2 you are well along in your journey to fight burnout and to be joyful as a healthcare provider. In this next section we will address the disease that is killing healthcare and how to respond.

The Disease Killing Healthcare

Our healthcare system is too expensive, millions are unable to access it because of the expense, quality is deteriorating, and in many cases, we're not getting what we pay for. Many healthcare providers are burned out, devalued, and no longer want to be in their job.

So, you may be wondering: How in the heck did we get ourselves in such a mess? In the greatest country in the world who spends the most on healthcare and is regularly bragging on how great it is, what happened?

Experts and pundits alike tout a litany of reasons. Increasing life expectancy, our reliance on sophisticated and expensive diagnostic tests and treatments, the costs of Big Pharma, duplication of care, fraud and abuse—the list goes on. Although these are all important contributors, none of them points to the underlying disease that's killing healthcare.

The Greed Virus

The healthcare system in some respects is like the human body. It has seven systems, and the health and survival of each is largely dependent on the health of the others, much like the inter-dependent relationship of the organs of the human body. For example, if your liver or kidneys fail, your body's health is severely impacted, even if your heart and lungs are functioning normally.

The seven systems of healthcare include the patients, the physicians and other providers, hospitals, third-party payers, the manufacturers of drugs and equipment, the legal profession, and the government. For the body of healthcare to be healthy, all seven systems must be in order.

The fundamental problem with American healthcare is that its seven systems are infected with the greed virus. Yes, the disease killing healthcare is greed, and it has infected people and corporations. A rapidly spreading infection of greed, entitlement, and unrealistic expectations. Unfortunately, it's human nature.

For decades, each system has been taking as much as it can, as fast as it can, and its insatiable greed has spread out of control. It's not sustainable.

Insurance companies raise premiums by double digits while denying coverage. The pharmaceutical companies charge astronomic prices for insulin, chemo-therapy, and many other life-giving drugs. Attorneys win multi-million-dollar settlements and drive regulatory costs skyward. Hospitals make millions while hiring less qualified nurses. Government officials swayed by corporate lobbyists tout that they care about the cost of healthcare. Physicians commoditize patients by performing unnecessary tests and procedures. And patients want perfect healthcare and they want it now. Everyone's been taking, and the system is dying.

The body of healthcare is desperately ill and it represents one of the most important societal issues of our day. Greed is the fundamental problem and it's driving up costs, driving down quality, and burning out its providers. And as it did in the greed-infected financial and banking industry, the system is destroying itself.

This is what happens when you commoditize healthcare and stray too far from its fundamental role in society. Healthcare is a basic need of every human being. But when healthcare becomes a commodity, the greed virus spreads, the end user suffers, the body dies, while the greediest make millions.

Potentially lethal, the greed virus must be brought under control. The health of the body of healthcare and our nation depends on it. And with the majority of us sharing some culpability, we're all responsible for its treatment and solution. We're all responsible for the health of the nation.

Solutions

In the next several chapters, we'll explore the greed virus and how it infects each system in the body of healthcare. The goal here is not to finger-point or to cast judgment. The goal is to identify the issues and how greed-associated behavior negatively impacts physician happiness and causes burnout. As is the case with nearly all viruses, there is no cure or quick fix. But once identified, we can then offer solutions and survival tactics to effectively manage the virus, reducing burnout and finding joy.

CHAPTER 14

THE PHYSICIAN GREED VIRUS: KEEP LOOKING UP

Sitting in my daughter Lindsey's school auditorium, the headmaster welcomed in the incoming students and parents. Mr. Grant was sharing with us his experience the year prior with one of his athletes on the boys' varsity soccer team.

Clearly passionate, Mr. Grant wanted to emphasize some of the values many of the students were learning as part of their maturing process.

The soccer game was close, sudden death, and the rivalry between the two teams intense. His star forward Kingsley had not scored and was getting beaten down by his defensive opponent. The other player, highly skilled in game and tactics, was fouling him unfairly, landing some pretty good punches, always under the radar of the referee.

Nearing the sidelines, frustrated, Kingsley repeatedly cried out, "Coach Grant, I can't take it. I can't take his elbows and punches any longer. I've got to fight back."

Quietly, with arms firmly crossed, Coach responded, "No, you won't, Kingsley, no you won't. You're different."

"But coach, we've got to win! He's cheating."

Coach repeated, "No, you're different."

In the midst of the turmoil, the player had an epiphany. "You're right, Coach, I am different." More determined than ever, Kingsley played on.

It's funny how an epiphany—an aha moment—often occurs with small everyday occurrences or experiences that changes the current situation and perhaps one's future.

Kingsley was reminded that he was different. He wasn't going to react and fight. He wasn't going to break the rules. He was going to honor the game, his coach and team, and most importantly himself. Because he was different.

I believe when Kingsley walked off that field at game's end, when he was showering later, hurting and bruised, and even today when he remembers that game, he's proud of himself. He didn't cheat. He didn't sacrifice his integrity. He swallowed his pride and pushed beyond his fear of losing. He chose not to respond, knowing that he could. He was looking up to his mountaintop.

The Physician Greed Virus

I believe that many physicians are infected with the greed virus, and it predisposes them to burnout. **The infection presents differently with varying signs and symptoms. Greed, inflated pride and identity, and fear are common manifestations.** Some demonstrate a personality flaw or tendency. In others, there are those who conduct some pretty significant unfavorable actions and behaviors. Fortunately, its adverse effects and spread are limited by our transcendent or internal compass—our immune system fighting the virus.

It's important to know how much greed is contributing to burnout. The greed virus is not curable, but many of its symptoms can be minimized. Recognition of the diagnosis and its effects can be healing and beneficial. With wisdom, we can adapt and be more fulfilled even with our weaknesses, all important in battling burnout.

Financial Pressure

Physicians are under increasing financial pressure compared to years gone by. Our declining income in the face of rising costs is only worsening. The lifestyle we've become accustomed to, and which some feel entitled to have, is becoming a fading reality.

For those who witnessed the last two or three market crashes, living the good life while simultaneously saving enough to ensure a similar lifestyle in retirement is challenging. And in the excitement of high-paying positions at tech companies, start-ups, and the financial industry, it's obvious that our position in the white-collar food chain has been diminished.

Our lifestyle, expectations, security, and ego are all being threatened or diminished. As a result, many have placed themselves under too much financial pressure to compensate and are working harder. Running harder and faster year after year is stressful and invites burnout.

Greed

Superimposed on this financial stress, greed adds fuel to the fire. It's fair to say that most of us are infected to varying degrees with the greed virus. It's just human nature.

Greed is an intense desire or longing for material gain, be it food, money, status, or power. It's when your thoughts, actions, and behaviors become unhealthy or detrimental as a result of an unquenchable appetite for temporal things, not transcendent. There's nothing wrong with wanting nice things and security, but there's a fine line between that and greed.

There's a fine line between working hard for reward, and sacrificing yourself and others for money. There's a fine line between establishing a sensible 401(k) and an endless yearning for more. It's prudent to run a successful business, but some physicians cross the line for profit.

Greed is insidious. It escalates as wealth increases. It's often justified by earned wisdom or entitlement. It's much more common in physicians than they would like to think.

The virus of greed drives us to overbook clinics and surgical schedules. It pushes us to hire less-skilled staff who can therefore be paid less, shifting the burden and frustration of our operations to us. It's why some have dumbed down their medical records to cut-and-paste templates, sacrificing their own excellence and personal satisfaction.

As the greed virus spreads, so does its adverse effects. Temptation lures us to make fewer mountaintop decisions and encourages unhealthy actions and behavior that negatively impacts healthcare.

Negative decisions like seeing more than fifty patients a day, processing them through like cattle. The excessive ordering of lucrative tests and procedures. Over-billing Medicare, and recommending surgery that's not indicated.

Unfortunately, some physicians' behavior is driven by greed.

I recently asked a friend who works with physicians what he felt was our fundamental weakness or character flaw. His calm response, "You guys don't care like you pretend you do. Too many physicians think more about themselves than their patients. I mean, just look at the crap some of you guys do." An interesting comment from one of the finest men I know.

I'm not here to finger-point or to cast judgment. But if you're not joyful in practicing medicine, perhaps you've crossed the line and have become infected with greed. On one side is joy, purpose, and fulfillment. On the other side, it's not.

Whether or not you're financially successful, I don't believe these actions and behavior are nourishing and fulfilling. No matter how much money you have, you cannot fool your soul. Gordon Gekko was wrong: greed is not good. Greed erodes. Greed promotes burnout.

Inflated Pride and Identity

While discussing the content of my book, a colleague of mine reminded me of the seven deadly sins: Pride, greed, lust, envy, gluttony, wrath, and sloth, each thought to be excessive extensions or abuses of one's natural passions or tendencies.

As the greed virus spreads, it also manifests as inflated pride and identity. Pride, in and of itself, is not bad. We should be proud of ourselves and accomplishments. We should be especially proud of helping and serving others. However, when pride distorts into overconfidence, like, "I'm always right; I'm better than others"—that is destructive.

I have mixed feelings when it comes to pride and how it applies to burnout. Every provider wearing the three-quarters-length white lab coat—our suit of armor—needs to be proud of themselves. Being confident and assured is an integral part of your joyfulness and survival. The weight of serving others rests on those straight shoulders; pride makes them stronger and able to bear the responsibilities.

But I think that many of us infected with the greed virus become too prideful. Exaggerated pride correlates with an inflated self-image. Our sense of identity becomes too narrowly defined by what we do, rather than who we are. Our accomplishments and status feed our inflated identity and ego, but neither provides happiness and meaning.

To some degree, it's no wonder our identity is inflated. Being identified as a physician separates us in the eyes of many. Medical students are often held up on pedestals and treated differently by parents, friends, romantic partners, and even strangers. Even among lay persons, other professionals, and others who serve, I think many look at physicians as being different.

But ask any doctor's child who's had to deal with that absent seat in the crowd at their recital, that missed birthday or Thanksgiving, that garage door waking them late at night—are all rationalized by the MD identity. **The problem with inflated pride and identity is that it promotes undesirable behavior and fosters physician burnout. In many respects we may be responsible for our own problems.**

It's the physician with inflated pride and identity who berates a nurse in the operating room, who doesn't respect the administration or the hierarchy, who consciously or subconsciously believes that they're better and smarter. Physician group decision-making is nearly impossible because "I'm always right." And infected with inflated pride and identity, a physician thinks about that ungrateful or unreasonable patient: "It's my way or the highway; I hold all of the cards."

These thoughts, actions, and behaviors are accompanied by stress, anger, lack of contentment, and a chronic case of thinking that "every day is a bad one." There's a strong possibility you may be disliked or not respected by others, and unless you're narcissistic, your body and soul may not like you either.

When you put so much emphasis on being a physician versus being a parent, a friend, a community builder, a good steward of your health, it does propose an important question: What happens when the profession of medicine and being a physician lets you down?

Your inflated identity would then deflate. Deflation leads to frustration, anger, and meaninglessness. Burnout.

Fear

Greed and inflated pride and identity predisposes human beings to becoming fearful. Fear is a feeling of perceived danger or threat, closely related to anxiety, stress, panic, and sadness.

Many of us are fearful about living a lower standard of living, either now or in retirement. Or we are fearful that we really can't afford that second home, that private university for our child, that annual vacation. What would my friends, my neighbors, my family, or worse—my entitlement and ego—think if they only knew my financial reality?

In the new commoditized world of healthcare, I think many of us are fearful of no longer being top dog. No longer being a highly respected and envied pillar in our society. No longer calling the shots as king or queen of our own private-practice domain.

Instead, we are now an employee, a cog in the wheel, our job relegated to "provider," serving customers and making them satisfied. We have handed over our precious autonomy and control to consultants and administrators, which is a true shot over the bow to our power and ego.

Many of us are fearful of slowing down if we make healthy work and life decisions. All of which might be necessary to give ourselves the margin and the balance we need to fight burnout and find joy.

Instead, we push even harder to keep the status quo longed for by our greed, inflated pride and identity, and fear. Ask yourself: *Where is it going to end?*

Addressing the Virus

Addressing one's personal greed virus is integral to successfully winning the battle against burnout. Greed, along with inflated pride and identity, and fear all must be addressed in order to find joy and fulfillment.

Let me share with you a few recommendations.

Realize Your Journey

First and foremost, it's imperative to believe in your journey to live on your mountaintop and finish strong. Realize and accept the difficult, challenging, but rewarding steep ascent to the summit. Imprint this calling into your soul, and into your daily thoughts and actions.

Think it. Write it down. Say it out loud over and over. And start climbing.

Shed the Heavy Pack

It's so important in making the climb to the summit to lighten your load. Lighten that heavy pack that's weighing you down and pulling you back down into the valley of burnout.

Unfasten the straps and shed the heavy pack of greed, inflated pride and identity, and fear that hinders you from climbing effectively. The arrogance that keeps you caught in the past and prevents you from change. It takes a lot of self-realization, but only you know how tight those straps are really tied.

It's a fine line between successfully climbing and falling back into the valley. The key to success is to keep looking up. Keep looking up toward your transcendent or internally driven purpose, your calling, the one that's imprinted in your soul that drives the difficult climb and journey.

Through medical school and residency, we are driven by testing achievements, awards, and academic accolades. When we finally enter the real world there are no more tests, no more grades. Only money serves as the universal value system for our society. But in the context of medical care, if we default to money as our value system, we find ourselves in a shallow, empty, and ultimately dark place. We have to redefine and reclaim a higher value system, our mountaintop.

Kingsley the soccer player had shed his heavy pack of inflated pride and fear of losing the game. He subscribed to a higher value system that made him invincible.

Choose Not To

Resist sacrificing eternal things for temporal ones. What I've come to realize is that strength, wisdom, and meaning are fostered by knowing you can do something, but choose not to.

Know you can see more patients and work longer hours but choose not to. Know you can aggressively bill third-party payers, but choose not to. Know you can reprimand the nurse in the operating room, but choose not to.

The result: fist pumps congratulating self-control and discipline, truly promoting personal pride and strength. Prioritizing what's good and right, you find yourself more content and living closer to your summit. The "choose not to" will make you a better climber, enabling you to battle the greed virus and burnout.

Like Kingsley after the game, feeling proud and strong, knowing he could punch back but chose not to, you too can persist beyond greed, inflated pride and identity, and fear.

Listen To . . .

So, how do you know when you're starting to slip and fall back into the valley? *Listen to your internal compass, your conscience.* You can't fool your inner self, the differentiator between right and wrong.

When you find yourself rationalizing your actions, and even your thoughts regarding a particular person or situation, I suggest a pause. Self-justification is often your conscience speaking. It's sending you a signal that needs to be heard.

An effective climber trusts their wits, hands, and footing. These are all finely-tuned instruments to detect unsure or risky steps. With eyes fixed upward, they ascend one step at a time. Similarly, we must trust our transcendent and internal purpose. We must listen to our calling's voice, our conscience. Our conscience is the instrument guiding us upward, one solid step at a time.

Resist flirting with unsure footing and becoming desensitized to missteps and bad behavior. Resist doing what others around you justify as normal and acceptable:

- "It's what the patient or referring physician expects or wants."
- "Nowadays, you have to play the game."
- "I don't do that procedure; it doesn't reimburse enough."
- "I'm working eighty hours a week to accommodate the patients!"

All these narratives justifying missteps are common. Narratives that blame others and not ourselves. This was once foreign to our profession, but now is ingrained dogma. Accepted, but sadly, self-destructive.

Yes, listen to your narratives. Listen carefully. Explore them for evidence of infection with greed, inflated pride and identity, and fear.

And if infected, realize your journey, shed the heavy pack, choose not to, and listen to your internal compass and narratives. Renew your thinking. Trade destructive narratives and beliefs with those more closely aligned with your mountaintop.

The higher you climb, the greater the enrichment and fulfillment. The higher you ascend, healthier thoughts and narratives will make you a better climber. **At higher altitudes, the views of meaning and joy are more spectacular. Most importantly, keep looking up; the ascent to the summit is difficult but well worth it.**

Remember that you are different and have been called to climb. Win, lose, or draw, live on your mountaintop, and finish strong.

Team Talk

It's difficult for some nurses and advanced practice providers to work in an environment shaped by physicians infected with the greed virus. A physician's actions, words, and philosophy can permeate the culture, adversely affecting all. Provider joy and fulfillment is sometimes jeopardized, and burnout increases.

Being asked to work harder and to do more tasks is stressful, especially if you feel underappreciated or inadequately compensated. Performing questionably indicated procedures and tests, or witnessing unsatisfactory care, is discouraging. And when you stop respecting or believing in the mission of the workplace, your soul feels empty.

The physician greed virus and how it affects other providers is a complex issue with no simple solutions. People's behavior inherently has many shades of gray and how it's interpreted by others varies. Let me provide you with three strategies that you may find beneficial if you're not seeing eye to eye with your physician.

First, accept that there will always be players in life who may cross the line and not play a fair game. Many of the worst offenders are often popular, and at first glance seem noble.

By looking up you can focus on your mission to be an excellent player and to help others. By looking up you can make mountaintop decisions that nourish and inspire yourself to reach the summit.

Second, remember that you are different. You are armed with love and compassion, and have been called to use your gifts and talents to serve. Ignore the playing conditions and narrow your focus to your relationship with patients. And at day's end, even if you sometimes are hurt and bruised, you can recall the day and be proud of yourself.

Third, sometimes a different game needs to be played. Don't be afraid to move on to better fields if your working environment is unhealthy or unacceptable. Don't sacrifice your personal health and joy, but instead make the right choice for you and find new employment. Remember our manager's wise words: "This is a job and not your life."

Nurses and APPs can also be infected with the greed virus. Their greed, inflated pride and identity, and fear can adversely affect them and promote burnout. To those people, I hope that the advice provided in this chapter is beneficial. I encourage them to do the Journey Moment exercise.

A JOURNEY MOMENT

Do you believe that some of your thoughts, words, and actions are a result of greed, inflated pride and identity, and fear? If yes, write down one example.

_____

_____

_____

_____

_____

_____

Do you think what you identified predisposes you to more frustration and burnout? If yes, how?

_____

_____

_____

_____

Is there one thing you could shed from your heavy pack to address this issue and make your life and career more enjoyable?

_____

_____

_____

_____

_____

Along the same line of thinking, what is one thing you are doing that if you chose not to do, it would make you feel less stressed and more fulfilled?

_____

_____

_____

_____

What is one rationalization or narrative that relates to this issue that you should listen to that would bring you one step closer to your mountaintop?

_____

_____

_____

_____

Take a break. Then write down a second thought, word, or action and redo the above exercise. Keep a journal or use the space provided. Expand on it. Read it over and over. You are on a journey to change your life by addressing your biggest challenge—your own greed virus. Good luck.

CHAPTER 15

MY BLACK OLIVES AND ANCHOVIES:
THE HEALTHCARE INSURANCE INDUSTRY

Kettle-cooked barbecue chips, all-meat pizza, spicy red sauce, a burger, scallops—I absolutely love food, and the list of foods I love is seemingly endless. Once nicknamed "Scottie the Wonder Hog" for my regular over-indulgences, I think I can generally out-eat most people (except for my best friend Johnny).

However, I cannot stand black olives and anchovies. I would never put one of them into my mouth. I can't even write about them without grimacing.

Similarly, the healthcare insurance industry puts a bad taste in my mouth. Like black olives and anchovies, my distaste for them is visceral.

I think when it comes to physician burnout and any blame we might cast toward corporatized healthcare, I cannot think of any other entity that causes more harm to providers and patients than the healthcare insurance industry.

I see patients suffering financially and medically on a daily basis as a result of third-party-payer corporate greed. It saddens me. Physicians and nurses are endlessly beaten down by rules, regulations, and lower reimbursements rigged to maximize corporate profits at our expense. And their insane premiums and deductibles now threaten the financial health of so many. The healthcare insurance industry greed virus is spreading without conscience, hurting millions.

Posting billions of dollars in net earnings, insurers typically have similar amounts stowed in reserve to cover that rare worst-case scenario. It's difficult to judge whether such financial success is appropriate or fair, but it's troubling knowing they do so at the expense of patients and others. They deny coverage of medications. They refuse to pay for life-saving scans and surgeries recommended by physicians. Let's face it: they make millions by playing doctor.

The insurance industry has a tremendous conflict of interest, and I believe it's rigged when it comes to paying claims and providing you the service you hired them for. Patients pay their rate for the agreed upon coverage, but the insurance industry does everything possible not to deliver. Many actually incentivize their employees not to cover medical claims and services. It's somewhat of a misnomer to call them third-party payers, when they try so hard to be third-party non-payers.

And if I have to endure one more TV ad tagline touting how patient-centric the insurance industry is, I'll scream! Cheering patients on to live wonderful lives while at the same time significantly raising premiums and ruthlessly denying care. Why in America do we let them get away with this?

Generational Consequences

It's probably fair to say that most people are living month-to-month with their income and have very little financial margin for any larger expenses that may arise. When insurance premiums and deductibles increase, there's often that much less for food, gas, and other household expenses. Tough choices need to be made about balancing limited funds with bills and family needs.

Unlike the rising price of automobiles, homes, and many commodities, healthcare is a basic need and there's no other lower cost alternative. As its cost escalates, the average American not only has less money for their expenses, they have less available to save for college and retirement, let alone financial emergencies like job layoffs or illness.

The result is resorting to less expensive, unhealthier food choices in an already obese and diabetic population. This will have generational consequences. It results in less money for higher education in an already arguably less-educated country, which will have generational consequences. And less money saved for retirement will increase financial dependence on our economically strapped government, and will also have generational consequences.

With more people being unable to afford those rising premiums and deductibles, many face financial peril if and when they become sick. Without coverage, many avoid seeking medical attention, often gravely affecting their care. Untreated diabetes and hypertension, blood in the stool from an undiagnosed cancer, unaddressed swollen extremities from fluid soon to incapacitate the heart—this is now becoming our healthcare reality as more and more hard-working Americans cannot afford healthcare.

Eventually, someone has to pay. And trust me, placing the burden on government or on a small minority of others will negatively impact all.

Ruthlessness

The healthcare insurance industry and Medicare is financially destroying private physicians, making our lives miserable and promoting burnout. They pay us shamefully low reimbursements relative to the cost of delivering care, give us rules and regulations designed only so that they don't have to pay us, and set up one roadblock pre-authorization after another. We're forced to hire an increasing number of staff in an attempt to abide by their rules and survive as a small business, which is a losing battle. Our cries for help go unnoticed.

With Napoleon-like ruthlessness, insurers are relentless, taking our last dollars of profit and multiplying it into millions for themselves. This is an insatiable greed virus.

Insurance costs are out of control. Quality of care is being negatively impacted. Physicians are being forced out of private practice. Perhaps you're wondering how the insurance industry has managed to have such a negative impact on the body of healthcare? The simple answer: lobbyists.

The healthcare insurance industry accounts for one of the greatest shares of lobbyist spending by any industry. Their lobbyists spend millions on politicians, who then pass legislation that favors the insurance industry. Your local congress representative and senators are well aware of what's happening regarding the healthcare insurance industry because they're in on the deal. A friend of mine from India once wisely stated, "America is the greatest democracy in the world that money can buy." It's sad, but it's true.

How do these companies rationalize such corporate greed that adversely affects so many? What's actually said in boardrooms as they plan out their next victim? Who will they deny care for this week? What physician group will they financially ruin, driving them out of private practice? What will their next advertising slogan promise in a hypocritical way?

Forgive me for my candor. And I do respect disagreement and opposing opinions. But thinking of their ruthlessness and greed, the healthcare insurance industry truly is my black olives and anchovies, and my distaste for them is visceral. Having said that, there is plenty of hope for all of us. Please read on.

TEAM TALK

The greed virus infecting the healthcare insurance industry and Medicare adversely effects nurses and APPs. When employers are paid less while simultaneously being bombarded by more regulations and skyrocketing overhead, it's more difficult to provide salary increases and bonuses to staff. The entire system becomes stressed.

Asking nurses to work harder without financial benefit eventually discourages and builds bitterness and resentment. The healthcare team becomes fractionated and loses harmony. Even the most loyal providers begin looking for more highly paid and less stressful opportunities.

The burdensome pre-authorizations, the rules and regulations and their associated tasks are killing our nurses. They are frustrated and demoralized by endless clerical duties and miss caring for patients. "I didn't sign up for this when I became a nurse," they often say.

Many nurses are leaving the profession, and job-hopping has become the new norm. But the greed virus of the healthcare insurance industry and Medicare does not care. Wall Street and lobbyists win, and continue to rule the day.

A JOURNEY MOMENT

Do you believe that the healthcare insurance industry and Medicare has contributed to physician burnout?

_____

_____

_____

_____

_____

_____

If yes, do you believe that physicians share any responsibility for allowing it to happen? If so, how have they?

_____

_____

_____

_____

_____

_____

CHAPTER 16

SUCCESSFULLY BATTLING THE HEALTHCARE INSURANCE INDUSTRY GREED VIRUS

How do we fight burnout and find joy in the midst of the healthcare insurance industry greed virus?

Remember your mountaintop. Remember that one of your most important survival tactics in battling burnout is to take ownership and accept the world of healthcare we now find ourselves in. Being angry and blaming others is not a good strategy. Look up and make mountaintop decisions that equip you to make the difficult ascent to the summit.

The insurance industry issue is a difficult one, but let me provide you with a few fist pump opportunities. In addition to the endless processes and expert staff you already have hired to deal with payments and third-party payers, the following suggestions may help you in fortifying the homeland.

A Culture of Excellence

In my practice, in support of our team's culture of delivering patient-centric excellence, we accept the need for pre-authorizations as a necessary cost of doing business.

We will not sacrifice quality only to lessen the clerical burden on my staff and myself. Giving in to the insurance industry negatively impacts patients and is demoralizing to providers. We are proud to assist our patients, and this healthy pride benefits our team. It's noteworthy how a simple change in mindset can make such a big difference.

Whether you like it or not, the need for pre-authorizations is here to stay, and likely will only increase. And battling the insurance industry with a heart of frustration, anger, and bitterness is not helpful. Instead, it's a regular reminder that standing for excellence is rewarding.

Yesterday I saw a patient I'm treating for urinary incontinence and she had had failed on a number of medications and another treatment. She tried a new pill, and has since been completely dry. Initially her monthly out-of-pocket expense for this new pill was $500 and was therefore unaffordable. After resubmitting her paperwork twice and persistence by my wonderful nurses, the drug was finally approved by her third-party payer, and she now pays less than $50. She gave me a hug for our efforts on her behalf; she is so grateful. And when I walked down the hall afterward to thank my team, the fist pumps were flying.

Empowerment

My staff are empowered to make decisions and to navigate the world of third-party payers without asking me for approval every step of the way. They fill out forms, call payers and patients. My job, in most cases, is only to provide my signature.

I've set up protocols allowing nurses and triage to call in generic prescriptions if and when step-therapy or other is required. Other than a nurse progress note, it all happens pretty seamlessly and under the radar.

In addition, staff are provided talking points to address common insurance issues. "I'm sorry. Dr. MacDiarmid doesn't make medication changes over the phone based on your insurance or co-pay. Unfortunately, we have too many requests and it's become overwhelming. Please call your insurance company and bring with you the medications they cover with their co-pays. Bring it to your next visit, or if needed, we can schedule you for an earlier appointment."

The immediate result of empowering and instituting such simple narra-

tives is improved efficiency, happier staff, and less repetitive stress and frustration. Less burnout.

Empower others to complete forms like family leave, workers' compensation, and return-to-work correspondence, as you know these forms seem endless. Develop a system in which your signature is generally all that's required. Stop shouldering the multiplying tasks that are weighing you down.

Pick Your Time

Fortunately, as a voiding dysfunction subspecialist, my need for peer-to-peer reviews with insurance companies seeking approval for tests or surgery is rare. In contrast, my oncology partner is heavily burdened, and his frustration is sometimes palpable. He just wants to be left alone to practice literature-based medicine.

Not having lived in my partner's shoes, perhaps a minor suggestion for those burdened by too many peer-to-peer reviews is to pick your time when you have to do these annoying tasks. Put them all together in a one-time bucket and use your staff to organize the connection between the two parties. Shouldering a frustrating call during an already stressful day or when you're tired is not recommended. If resubmitting templates and medical records justifying care don't suffice, then at least have the peer-to-peer during a non-stressful time, or better still, at day's end on speaker phone when you're driving home to be with family.

Look in the Mirror

If only I had a dollar for every time I blamed the insurance industry for causing my woes about practicing medicine, or got up on a soapbox on how the free market of supply and demand doesn't apply to physicians. But I've learned blaming others doesn't help.

Much like what we discussed in promoting healthy communication in fortifying the homeland, it's helpful once again to look in the mirror and redefine the problem. You'll realize that you may be partially culpable.

How we can finger-point and feel sorry for ourselves if we're not willing to fight? When we're not willing to stand up and say no? When clearly we don't have a red line that can't be crossed, our futile attempts of resistance is laughable.

Without a red line, surgery is now reimbursed at a fraction of what it was two decades ago. Without a red line, 30 percent of personnel in a physician's office are hired purely for paperwork, and never actually engage in patient care. Unwilling to say no, charting requirements are out of control, pre-authorizations are endless, and next year's raise is possibly minus 2 percent. And now, seemingly too late to say no, the majority of physicians have surrendered and are now owned by healthcare systems. This is an unbelievable mess, arguably self-inflicted by the top 1 percent.

So, why no red line? Not surprisingly, we most commonly tout patient care. With patients caught in the middle, saying no could jeopardize us looking after them. And though we should be proud of our patient-centric stance, I suggest other reasons in addition.

In the mirror, I see the reflection of pride, greed, and even fear. Yes, I believe that our own greed virus is somewhat responsible for our inability to define a red line and to say no.

Many physicians are unwilling to say no because we're afraid to risk short-term financial health to ensure long-term security. Unwilling to say no as a unified voice, some physicians are more interested in self-preservation. Perhaps we are too proud or too divided to speak up and expose the greed virus of third-payer payers, and our lobbying dollars may be too miniscule relative to theirs. It is actually illegal for physicians to strike, but there is more to it than that.

Those of us in the profession of medicine are not unified in our voice and actions. We are weak and divided by pride, greed, and fear. The profession of medicine is too weak to fight. And trust me, our adversaries know it.

In turn, we trade saying no to third-party payers for working harder, shifting income streams to ancillaries, and for some, breaking rules and misbehaving. And with fewer places left to hide, one day all physicians may be working for CEOs of healthcare systems. A sad ending to never drawing a red line.

But in spite of it all, taking responsibility and accepting our inability to define our red line is an important, actionable step in fighting burnout and finding joy. Less finger-pointing reduces anger and stress. Remember, sharing some of the blame, oddly, is a solution to personal torment. Perhaps accepting and learning from the school of hard knocks might reveal the path to a brighter future.

Stop Looking

When it comes to third-party payers and what we receive in reimbursement, stop looking. Relative to the cost of overhead, looking at it is likely to frustrate, irritate, anger, or worse. Although it's tempting, this worry may lure you away from patient-centric and literature-based medicine, none of which will help your burnout.

Instead, keep looking up. Clothed in your suit of armor, believe that excellence and doing the right thing for patients will win the day. **Practicing without thinking about reimbursement is so much less stressful.** Take care of patients, and everything else will take care of itself.

As a physician, never discuss finances with your patients. Leave these discussions to your expert staff. Your focus is on excellence and patient care. Trust me, when dollars are spoken by providers, misinterpretation is rampant. Money tarnishes a caring patient-physician relationship.

Make Peace with the Enemy

Benefits can come from speaking with third-party payers to negotiate win-win opportunities. Insurance companies are well aware that their premiums are becoming untenable, and are starting to look for lower cost opportunities.

Strong-armed by healthcare systems that demand astronomical prices, they know that independent physicians can deliver much more efficient and less expensive care.

Many physician-owned surgical centers are now negotiating bundled payments with third parties, rightfully boasting about lower costs, high patient satisfaction, and arguably higher quality than hospitals. Some friends of mine in private practice have negotiated a fair price for in-office procedures that benefits all—including the patient. And perhaps with negotiations and making peace with the enemy, we can minimize or eliminate many of the pre-authorizations and rules burdening us all.

So, where do we go from here? In the midst of the healthcare insurance industry greed virus, my black olives and anchovies, I suggest: focus on excellence, empower your staff, pick your time, look in the mirror, stop looking at line-by-line finances, and make peace with the enemy.

All of this is a better diet to fight burnout and to find joy.

TEAM TALK

Let me provide a number of ways to help nurses and APPs feel more fulfilled and help fight burnout in the midst of third-party payer greed.

Try Not to Compromise

Try not to compromise your standards when caring for patients. Provide the care that you would want for yourself and your loved ones. Fight for the pre-authorization of the medication that worked for them, and realize the importance of completing their family leave form in a timely fashion. Your pride in knowing you fought and won a battle for a patient will empower and reward you.

Be Efficient

As discussed, develop skills and techniques that will make you more efficient in answering tasks and performing clerical duties. Become a better fighter with a mindset that you are willing to work hard, so long as you do not sacrifice your personal joy and health to accommodate the system.

Appreciate the Financial Reality

I empathize with providers who are frustrated by their compensation. But sometimes a better appreciation of your employer's financial reality can help reset expectations and bring some peace and acceptance.

The healthcare team must fight as one against the greed virus of third-party payers. In many cases, it's us against them and reinforcements are not on their way. But it's a battle that we must win. The health of the nation depends on it.

Be Cautious of Greener Pastures

Nurses are switching jobs at a record pace citing better working hours and less stressful conditions, but it's heavily based on healthy sign-on bonuses and higher wages. At first glance, who would blame them?

But be cautious moving to greener pastures especially if you like your teammates and current job. Most employers have plenty of openings, but there may be reasons why they are offering such a good deal.

An environment that nourishes you and one in which you believe in the mission of the organization will pay great dividends long-term. If you don't fit with the culture of your new employer, a higher income will likely not sustain you. Ask yourself why you enjoy your current job and what attracted you to it in the first place. The answer may grant you wisdom moving forward.

Advanced practice providers are similarly being tempted by economics to move on to greener pastures. I can understand their reasoning, but please be cautious. Physicians spend enormous time and treasure training APPs, and a history of frequent moves will likely be identified as a red flag.

A JOURNEY MOMENT

Do you think your happiness practicing medicine is adversely affected by your thoughts and interactions with third-party payers?

Is yes, can you think of a few strategies that would help you better adapt to the current environment? Write down at least one and how doing it might benefit you.

1. _____

2. _____

3. _____

Chapter 17

A Litigious America: Is this Really What We Want?

It was late afternoon, wrapping up day four of what was expected to be an exhausting five-day trial. We'd spent days listening to testimony and professional opinions. I was next up to bat, after months of preparation warming up in the bullpen as an expert witness. I sat watching the tired-looking jurors, and trying to keep still as I battled with my attention deficit disorder.

I was confident in my preparation, but I was still nervous at the thought of being drilled as an expert witness by the onslaught of curve balls, sliders, and yes, the high hard ones that I knew were going to be thrown my way by the fierce plaintiff attorney. Between you and me, this guy was tough, and it was obvious that this was not his first playoff game.

I'd been warned about his masterful skills and artistry in the courtroom. He had a unique ability to capture and influence his audience, especially the trusting souls inhabiting the jurors' dugout. He was a charismatic speaker, irritating, but somehow likeable. Oddly, in the midst of his near-perfect showmanship, like a nervous tic, he repetitively unbuckled and buckled his belt, tucking in his oversized, faded gray wrinkled shirt.

The lawsuit came as a result of a tragic ending to an otherwise routine operation on a beautiful young teen named Sarah. Just two years before her death, she had been sadly rendered paraplegic as a result of a motor vehicle accident. Unable to control her legs, bowel, and bladder, Sarah was admitted to the hospital because of a stone blocking the catheter that drained her bladder.

Admitted Saturday night by Dr. Kevin Franklin, the on-call urologist, he took her to the operating room the next morning, where he successfully removed the stone and changed her catheter. Following surgery, and after nearly six hours of routine recovery, she was discharged home to her mom's care—stable, smiling, and otherwise back to normal. Yet tragically and silently she died later that night. Before the clock struck midnight, her mother was screaming for help, unsuccessfully trying to resuscitate the lifeless Sarah.

Two and a half years later we were at the trial suing Dr. Franklin, his recovery nurse, and the hospital for medical malpractice. Following months of critical review of hundreds of pages of physician and hospital records, binders full of family testimonies and expert opinions, it was crystal clear to me that the defendants were innocent of all allegations. But that means little when it comes to proving lack of culpability in such an emotionally charged and tragic case.

Not only did Dr. Franklin and Jill meet the standard of care that in a fair-minded world would prove innocence, they went beyond the call of duty. I testified their medical care was absolutely superb and superior to that given by the majority of providers. Every *t* was crossed, every *i* dotted, their documentation was as clean as a whistle.

The hospital notes too sang out a melody of unconditional, loving care. (And unfortunately, this good old-fashioned kind of medicine is becoming a thing of the past.) All the positive cheerleading, that fresh glass of water, a few jokes repositioning her pillow, but most importantly, the extra time they provided Sarah.

There Were No Winners

"All rise." The jurors who looked like your neighbors entered and robotically took their seats. The judge wore a traditional black silk gown, and was tall and handsome. And just like on TV, we heard, "Introduce your first witness." The attorney stood. The stakes were high, the emotions intense. Observing from the outfield, concentrating on each and every word knowing its potential relevance, I was agitated by a recurring thought—there is so much sadness in the room, and in this game there are no winners.

Day after day, the courtroom presented a graveyard of souls covered by a blanket of senseless sorrow, each feeling wronged by the other. Anticipation high, people took sides, sitting in their small wedding-like groups on one side of the aisle or the other, and from time to time, each gazed over at their unknown but decided enemy. What a waste. So much sorrow. So much greed. All because of money, opportunity, or perhaps revenge.

Dr. Franklin had given twenty-nine years of unconditional love and excellence to help others. I liked the man, respected him, and identified with him immediately.

For days, though, he was maligned as an "uncaring hack" by the opposing team, and indirectly a murderer for his careless misconduct; the strikes were impressive. And at first glance, convincing. Unable to scream out and defend himself, I put myself in his shoes; my breaths quickened as I shed his tears, appreciating his misery.

Win, lose, or draw, this lawsuit was his last straw. Dr. Franklin had decided to quit medicine and retired months prior to the trial. He was scarred for life. What a way to end a lifelong commitment to caring.

His wife reminded me of my wife Andrea. In spite of her cheerleading smile, her pain and sorrow were deeply imprinted in her soft blue eyes. The sadness seemed to age her daily. Her smile was so brave as she frequently consoled her husband, rubbing his shoulders as he was being maligned by others. Their experts were taking no prisoners.

Nurse Jill seemed naïve to the court. She wept profusely, just feet from the jurors, as she was accused of neglecting Sarah and fraudulently changing the medical record to cover her tracks. It was a time-stopping moment. Tucking in his shirt, the plaintiff's attorney showed no mercy. "Ma'am, your late entry in the chart was a lie, wasn't it? Simply a lie, wasn't it?"

It was rough watching her sob, attempting to gather her thoughts and respond to his repetitive accusations and questioning. She was no match for the experienced interrogator. Under the circumstances she defended herself well and was believable. I was proud of her.

The blanket of sorrow did not spare anyone. The jurors who perhaps just wanted to get back to work or to go home to their friends and family weren't benefiting from this attempted slaughter of the reputations of a doctor and a nurse. The family, appearing poorer and less educated, likely did not understand the intricacies of the case; it must have been painfully frustrating.

The plaintiff "experts" were a sorry bunch. They were either stupid or liars, perhaps both. Like the plaintiff's attorney, they clearly were there for the money. Like him, they didn't care about the truth.

I snuck a glance at Sarah's mom, wondering what she was thinking. I can't imagine how she must have felt, and continues to feel to this day.

What was she thinking when the defendants, directed by a pair of brilliant, stern, but compassionate female defense lawyers protected the accused and set the record straight? What was she thinking when what we testified is not what her family's lawyer had told her?

Her baby was gone. Her baby died after routine surgery. Her baby who she tried to resuscitate. Something must have gone wrong and someone must be responsible. Someone is to blame, and someone must pay. She was the true victim, and it was awful. Only the truth comforts my pain for her sorrow. Unfortunately, Sarah died of a rare undiagnosed metabolic disorder which caused her to stop breathing several hours after anesthesia.

Perhaps I'm mistaken, but as I stood up to the plate, gently laying my hand on the leather Bible, I felt the plaintiff's attorney was concerned about my presence.

I feel sorry for the family, sorry for the hundreds of thousands of dollars spent by the insurance companies to protect their doctors, hospital, and staff.

I'm sorry for what society has become and how the greed virus of the medical legal profession is killing the body of healthcare and burning out physicians. It's a malicious virus destructive to all.

It was not my first playoff game either.

Yes, the truth won out and the defendants were found not guilty, but in this game, there were no winners.

Is This What We Really Want?

Blame, entitlement, and endless multi-million-dollar settlements all dim the sun shining on our wonderful nation.

We have engineered such an automatic shoot-from-the-hip response of holding others financially accountable if we feel that they've wronged us in almost any fashion. And we pass this pattern of thinking on to the next generation, each time becoming more ingrained and vindictive.

Our country was founded on forgiveness and tolerance, yet now blame and intolerance seem to rule the day. Once giving others the benefit of the doubt, we now live by an "It's your fault and you're going to pay!" mentality. Seeking legal counsel used to be a last resort, yet we now have a trigger-happy response, an actionable extension of our loss of civility. Of course, while this is a necessary function to protect the innocent, I argue this is only a cover story for the greed-infected litigation attorneys.

There are lawsuits for spilled hot coffee, no candy bars in prisons, fatigue in spin classes—the list is endless. We giggle at the ridiculousness, yet it does real harm. Corporations and businesses settle frivolous claims to safeguard brand image. Many people accused are unable to financially protect themselves. Too many are emotionally scarred from past litigation. We're all potential victims of often depraved individuals seeking financial compensation.

Representing one-sixth of our economy, healthcare has taken a direct hit from our litigious society, and is one of the most litigated and regulated industries. The resulting cost to the system and to each and every one of us is staggering. A recent report cited the annual cost of medical malpractice in the U.S. to be $55.6 billion, more than 2 percent of annual healthcare spending. Uncapped medical malpractice litigation added nearly $100 billion to the cost of hospital and physician services, and increased health insurance premiums by nearly 13 percent.

Physicians and hospitals have used and continue to use the threat of litigation to justify their over-prescribing of expensive tests, procedures, and surgery. The corpse of literature-based and common-sense medicine was buried years ago, and with many of us financially benefitting, few miss it. The public has become accustomed to such over-delivery of medical care and now demands it. Patients want perfect care, they want it now, and there's no turning back.

Whether you're for or against the liberal willingness to sue, it comes at a price: higher premiums and deductibles. Regulatory costs are skyrocketing. Medicare might soon be insolvent. Prices of drugs and care are ever-increasing. And with the stress and pressure associated with the fear of litigation, physicians are burning out and checking out.

The litigation greed virus is threatening the financial health of our nation, our healthcare system, and individuals. Like the courtroom, our nation is becoming a graveyard of souls covered by a blanket of senseless sorrow. With the virus being so destructive, is this really what we want?

Team Talk

I wonder how many nurses have ever thought of themselves having to sit in a courtroom and be questioned by a plaintiff attorney regarding the care they provided for a patient. It's a situation that most of them might never have imagined. One day they are doing bedside nursing, and the next placed under a microscope and accused of negligent behavior. It's a sad possibility to the millions of nurses who go to work each day to help others.

But unfortunately there are going to be more nurses wrongfully accused as the greed virus of litigation continues to spread and multiply. Advanced practice providers are also being sued at higher rates than ever before. With most providers now being employed by multi-billion-dollar healthcare systems, nurses and APPs have become bigger targets.

A Journey Moment

Do you believe that our litigious culture is negatively impacting healthcare and how it's delivered?

_____

_____

_____

_____

Do you believe that the fear of litigation is increasing physician burnout?

_____

_____

_____

_____

Does the litigious culture adversely affect you? If so, list three ways that it does.

1. _____

2. _____

3. _____

CHAPTER 18

THE EVER-PRESENT THREAT OF LITIGATION

A young partner of mine recently asked me for advice. He had just gotten off the phone with a patient's daughter who was upset about a complication her father had experienced following surgery. She was finger-pointing.

The complication was the one that urologists are most concerned about in undertaking that procedure. We highlight that complication to our patients when discussing the merits of it. It's one of the reasons why many urologists avoid performing that surgery. And if and when that complication happens, the consequences are not good.

Visibly shaken, my partner had handled the situation beautifully. His dialogue with the daughter, his documentation, his preoperative consent process—all were perfect.

It was obvious that he cared deeply. I saw it in his eyes and heard it in his concerned and saddened voice. It would be natural for him to second-guess himself. I've been there, I felt for him, and I reassured him.

It's the Environment

The adverse effects of litigation reach far beyond being sued.

The problem is not just litigation. The problem is the environment that the ever-present threat of litigation creates and promotes.

In the lifespan of a practicing physician, the likelihood of an actual lawsuit being brought is arguably low. But its looming threat significantly increases physician stress and promotes burnout.

The threat creates a stressful environment, an environment of pressure, anxiety, and fear. Mental fatigue from chronic worry and tension. Fatigue, frustration, over-documenting, over-checking, and the endless covering your butt with words, actions, and processes. Words, actions, and processes all done for the eyes of others, none that are adding to patient care or excellence.

These are stress and anxiety levels that go far beyond looking after the ill, the suffering, and those facing their own immortality. Because that is what we have trained for, what we thrive on, and for many of us, it's what makes us tick.

Instead, it's the unhealthy environment produced by litigation that is so endemic, so insidious, and always present. It almost becomes a part of our lifestyle.

Fingers Crossed

Opening an envelope from an attorney, the medical board, or even a patient, you just hope that there is not a problem. You get a request to send medical records to another entity, and for moments you wonder if the patient is upset. Noting that a nurse is having a lengthy call with a patient, you begin worrying that there's an issue. And weekly, when I'm walking down the hall with fingers crossed to examine a postoperative patient, Jenna gives me the thumbs-up signaling that all is okay, and I blow out an internal sigh of relief.

I've been practicing medicine for a long time, and this level of paranoia was not prevalent in my life just two decades ago. But things have changed. With an ever-increasing threat of litigation, I find myself crossing my fingers regularly.

Sticks and Stones

When it comes to the pressure of perfection in medicine, I believe there's no job more difficult than that of a surgeon. As mentioned, my surgical patients have high expectations, and they can be disappointed and upset when they are not met.

In spite of lengthy preoperative discussions regarding risks and benefits, there's very little tolerance among patients for poor outcomes or complications.

I've become accustomed to an interesting dynamic, one coined "the old switcheroo." This is a sudden unexpected variation or reversal, an act of intentionally or unintentionally swapping two objects. The old switcheroo is a seemingly odd expression to describe a patient-physician relationship, but the two objects switched in this case is the patient's assumed responsibility for their healthcare problem, and them then passing that responsibility on to their physician, especially following surgery. It's the oddest thing. The healthcare issue that they've had for years is now strangely the physician's doing if it's not cured by surgery. And if a complication occurs, it's the surgeon's fault. It's the transference of responsibility and blame.

Disappointed and upset patients can be rough in their language to you, and such talks are not recommended for the thin-skinned and naïve.

"I'm really disappointed in the outcome of your surgery. I think I'm worse. I wish I never had it. Your surgery messed me up."

"My wife's surgery was a complete waste of her time. All the money we spent. What happened? What went wrong? I thought you said it was just a simple outpatient procedure?"

Although there's the old adage, "Sticks and stones may break my bones, but words will never hurt me," I'm afraid for me, they do hurt.

I have given my life to helping others. Such words cut deeply. It's so discouraging and destructive. So difficult to forget. It's sometimes difficult to get up tomorrow to fight another day.

In a culture that devalues, blames, and discourages, it's difficult to resist bitterness, resentment, and disliking patients. Their conditional respect and affirmation based on outcomes is shallow. With limited tolerance for poor results and complications, tension grows, especially for surgeons.

We've Got Bleeding

Pressure, anxiety, and fear are commonly experienced by physicians when delivering healthcare that's invasive. A man's heart stops during an angioplasty for unstable chest pain. The patient develops an acute abdomen minutes after a colonoscopy. Those infamous words of a surgeon with sweat on her brow, "We've got bleeding." Yes, the practice of medicine is serious business, and it can be scary.

To the culture who demands perfection and takes it for granted, I ask: How would you like to be placing the paddles on a man's chest who just moments ago was enjoying life with his family? How would you like to be the physician calling the surgeon, telling him that you just perforated a patient's bowel removing a polyp? How would you like to be the one walking down the hall to relay to the family that their loved one bled to death during elective surgery?

Trust me, we physicians and other providers, inside our souls we too are bleeding from the seriousness of these circumstances. Bleeding, knowing we're responsible for its acute management and long-term sequelae. Bleeding, asking: did we do something wrong? We know that we're likely to be blamed, second-guessed, and even held accountable by others' thoughts, words, or actions. Blame is now endemic, and it causes so much worry and despair. It is hard enough to stand up and believe in yourself, and believe that you can help, that you could even cure. It is demoralizing when the patient-physician relationship starts with the threat of blame.

Going home with a bloodied suit of armor—this is when pressure, stress, and burnout prevails. Looking up to your mountaintop or asking a loved one for a hug might be a source of comfort.

We're Not Iron Man

A number of years ago, one of my best friends, David (alias Super D), and I were conversing about friendship and careers.

David has invented and modified a number of surgical procedures, and is respected internationally. I'm dead serious—he's a carbon copy of Robert Downey Jr. in *Iron Man*, with all his swagger and confidence. He's one of the smartest people I know, and I love him like a brother.

Standing waist-deep in the pool at a beautiful convention hotel in Nice, France, David said, "Scott, for years when I would enter the operating room I was pumped, I was ready. It was showtime." Tapping the water he continued, "I would actually play drums with my hands on the OR table once the patient was asleep. Nothing I couldn't do. Bring it on; I was fearless.

"Now, entering the room, I've not lost my skills, I still deliver excellent care, but my thoughts differ. I can't stop thinking about all the things that go can wrong, all the complications that can occur. You know the ones. Honestly, I just don't want to do this anymore."

One of the most destructive emotions that can overwhelm physicians associated with the culture of litigation is fear. Especially for surgeons and those performing invasive procedures. We experience fear-related stress and anxiety gnawing at our souls, keeping us awake at night, worrying. All of us are over-ordering tests, double-checking everything, and are now prisoners to the demands for perfection.

The primary source of fear is not the actual case or procedure. It's not the treatment or underlying diagnosis. The source of stress and anxiety is the fear of poor outcomes, of complications or missing something, and now in the world of commoditized healthcare, the fear of not reaching the "customer's" treatment goal and its downstream ramifications. The finger-pointing. The anger. The poor patient satisfaction score.

In addition to fostering stress and burnout, fear can negatively impact our function and performance. I call the functional decline that comes with it the "death spiral of avoidance."

We start avoiding difficult and risky cases. We avoid certain patient types and diagnoses. If there are fewer years remaining until retirement, we narrow our practice to routine cases, and off-load more difficult cases to younger partners. The irony is that more experienced surgeons have more training and skill to handle the complexities, but we may also be paralyzed by fear. We consciously or unconsciously change treatment algorithms, directing care away from stressors. Biased by fear and our attempts to reduce stress, we stop, we refer, we redirect, always supported by rationalizations.

But the death spiral and its negative effect compounds itself quickly. The more we avoid and stop doing, unfortunately, the more we lose our confidence. Now sidelined, we second-guess ourselves and start hiding even more from our job. Sadly, our surgical and technical skills quickly deteriorate. Some paralyzed by fear stop doing surgery altogether, and others retire earlier than planned.

Like a pitcher who gets the yips at the top of their game and starts throwing wild pitches, losing confidence is devastating. It's destructive to the individual and others counting on them, even career-ending. And no one is spared. Even Super D, the best of the best, can become fearful. Let's face it, we're not Iron Man.

Even the flirtation with going down this death spiral of avoidance scares me to this day.

Keep looking up. Keep doing those challenging cases. Our patients need our expertise.

TEAM TALK

The environment of pressure, anxiety, and fear created by the ever-present threat of litigation affects not only physicians but the entire healthcare team.

Nurses and APPs are living in a world of rules and regulations initially designed for patient safety, but now many exist to ward off the litigation greed virus. Patient care has been replaced by checking boxes on computers in order to meet requirements and to satisfy others. Less time at the bedside is threatening provider joy and limiting gratifying relationships with patients.

Providers are fearful of making mistakes or breaking a rule that may get them in trouble or even fired. They are stressed, caught in the middle between angry patients and their employer's philosophy of "the customer is always right." They have been stripped from making independent decisions, triaging even the simplest question to physicians.

Under the threat of litigation, the environment of healthcare has been sadly changed forever. It's no wonder provider burnout is everywhere.

A JOURNEY MOMENT

Do you get discouraged, stressed, mentally fatigued, or fearful as a result of the threat of litigation? If yes, list up to three ways that you're affected and elaborate on each.

1. _____
2. _____
3. _____

Would addressing some of your feelings and fears associated with litigious culture be beneficial to you? Please read on.

CHAPTER 19

FACING THE FEAR OF LITIGATION

Experts claim that the most effective way to deal with fear is to face it. To run toward it and not away from it. Action overcomes paralysis. Doing overcomes avoidance. Successfully dealing with fear despite a culture of litigation is essential to finding joy and fighting burnout.

When it comes to being a physician, you can't hide from the pressure, the responsibility; the list of the must-dos is endless. You can't hide from the risky cases, the unhappy patients, the letters from the medical board and attorneys. It's the environment; it's part of the job.

Resist trying to escape, because fear will always know where you're hiding. It will track you down and eventually defeat you. Being prepared for battle and protected by your suit of armor, facing and fighting your fear is the only successful strategy.

Because we live in an environment of litigation, let's talk about a number of ways to be better prepared for battle and to face our enemy. There are two important components: your mental strategies and your practical strategies.

Identify the Enemy

It's critical to identify the enemy that frightens you, that you're running away from or trying to hide from. Your technical skills, your confidence, adverse outcomes and sequelae, an unhappy customer, perhaps even failure. Be honest with yourself. You can't effectively fight a battle until you first identify the enemy.

Analyze the Battlefield

Analyze the battlefield and ask yourself the tough questions. Do you have a *skill* problem, or a *worry* problem? Have you lost your confidence, or are you trying to avoid risk and complications? Are you referring or unloading to others, not wanting to give the time and energy necessary to take on the task? Or perhaps it doesn't pay enough.

Only you can answer these questions. In the answer lies the solution as well as effective strategies.

Come Up with a Mental Battle Strategy

Lacking skills is arguably the easiest issue to contend with. Seek more training. Read. There are plenty of instructional videos out there. Attend online or live teaching courses and lectures. Remember that learning is what you're good at.

Don't be afraid to ask partners or other colleagues for assistance until you feel comfortable. Put ego aside because your noble goal to improve your skills is too important to waste. Relinquish your embarrassment; good partners will respect your transparency and be flattered by their opportunity to help. And don't be surprised when a partner becomes a friend in the process. Fist pump. That's priceless. They will join you on your path to the mountaintop.

The general surgeons in our hospital are excellent; I often refer to them as the Marines because they grind it out in the surgical trenches on a daily basis with so many sick people to contend with. For me, that would be taxing and stressful.

I recently asked one of the partners, Stephen, how the group handles their heavy acute surgical load, who are often high-risk and very ill patients.

He told me, "We always operate together. It makes a big difference. It improves care, reduces stress, and builds positive physician relationships. It's a great way to improve your skills, especially for us younger physicians. It may not be financially efficient, but it's definitely worth it."

Losing confidence can be devastating to a physician, and even worse for surgeons. I think one of the fastest ways to lose confidence is encountering a complication, especially if it's serious or you've experienced a string of complications within a short period of time. Complications should trigger a healthy reflection about the type of surgery that was recommended and the care delivered. In spite of providing excellent care, complications can really take the wind out of the sails of even highly experienced physicians.

A partner of mine recently had a pretty significant bleeding complication following a routine outpatient procedure that he performed. Having just graduated training, it set his confidence back a few steps. He paused, he second-guessed, he wondered. Unlike in his residency, the complication and its management and consequences rested solely on his shoulders.

While he could have gotten negative and discouraged, he fortunately chose a healthier mindset: he consciously chose to get back in the saddle as quickly as possible. He realized the importance of accepting the complication and continuing to move forward as a competent provider. Armed with self-reinforcement and confidence, he was ready to do a similar case again and did so successfully.

The death spiral of avoidance is incredibly destructive. Fearing poor outcomes and consequences is a slippery slope to paralysis. **One of the most effective ways to battle this fear is to stop thinking about yourself and circumstances, and instead think about the patient.**

When I think about the patient, their thoughts, their hopes, their vulnerability, it immediately brings me to a place of calm. I'm reminded that the patient is counting on me and my expertise. They need my help. They need my excellence. One human helping another. Immediately, I can feel the positive change in my thinking.

I trade worry about myself and fear of failure for straighter shoulders, knowing it's my responsibility to care for them. I trade a feeling of "I can't wait to finish this case" with "Let's make a difference to a fellow human being." I trade fear with "I'm proud to be a surgeon and I've got work to do." Let's face it, God granted the gift of surgery to just a small minority of the population. Like running to help someone in danger, that raw instinct to help another overrides any personal fear or concerns.

The environment of litigation and the practice of medicine often feels overwhelming when there's a complication, an angry phone call, a complaint from a patient. It can be unnerving. In the midst of work's already busyness, stress, and responsibility, these triggers can really add fuel to the fire.

Compartmentalize

When you're feeling overwhelmed, limit your thinking to the task at hand. Compartmentalizing thoughts is an effective way to reduce stress. As the circumstances become more overwhelming, narrow your focus even further, one step at a time, and you will negotiate the landscape.

The pager won't stop, the febrile patient in room one is short of breath, your wife is having a repeat mammogram. Many days with high levels of stress, it seems almost impossible not to feel defeated. But the skill of compartmentalizing is a winning strategy.

My buddy, Joe, a former Marine, told me that compartmentalization is referred to as "chow-to-chow" in basic training. In boot camp, the new recruits are often so beaten down by physical and mental stress, and so they are instructed to focus only on the immediate task. Their job is only to survive to the next meal, to the next chow. At times it seems impossible. But one meal at a time, they keep on going. Within a few weeks, the same hell becomes more tolerable.

During moments of stress when I feel that chow-to-chow may not be enough, I instruct Jenna that I don't want to be asked a question or bothered by any others, unless it's urgent, until things settle and my emotions normalize. At other times, I'll walk away. Don't underestimate the calm that a short time-out can bring to a stressful situation.

Reframe

Cognitive reframing is a technique used by therapists to help clients look at situations from a different perspective. It's a way of changing the way you look at something and, thus, changing your experience of it. Reframing refashions negative thoughts into positive ones, and thereby reduces stress and anxiety.

Stress can be triggered by events ranging from the annoying to the frightening, and can linger long after the event has passed. Too many days I'm feeling chronically annoyed, irritated, and frustrated, and pulled down into the valley of burnout.

Psychologists recommend becoming an observer and noticing your thoughts. Stand back and notice when your thoughts are becoming negative or stress-inducing. You must recognize your enemy in order to deal with it. Notice what's triggered your negative thoughts. Write them down. Journaling is a powerful tool for reducing stress.

As an observer, you become more mindful of your thinking and stressors. Detached, it's easier to observe unhealthy thoughts rather than remaining caught up in them. The lens through which you view the world changes, enabling you to reframe what you see and feel.

As you notice your negative thinking, ask yourself a number of questions. Are the things you're thinking really true, or are you being fooled by the past and by your emotions? Are there other ways to interpret the same triggers or circumstances? Are there different viewpoints that might serve you better? Challenge every negative thought and replace it with a more positive outlook. The results of reframing can be life-giving. We will speak more about reframing later on in the book when we talk about having a mind of a warrior.

Stop the Snowball

It's important to stop thoughts from snowballing when you're dealing with stress. Voicing to yourself or others, "The world's coming to an end!" is not beneficial. Allowing negative thoughts to snowball and escalate is destructive. Getting up on your soapbox, complaining, using biting sarcasm, and even anger are common and only make your burnout worse.

When such thoughts and words begin, stop the snowball. Immediately reframe and replace negative thoughts and words with positive ones. If needed, walk away from the stressor momentarily, because a time-out may be necessary.

Put each situation into perspective. Remind yourself that it can be handled, and it's not the end of the world. "This too shall pass" are generational words of wisdom that can be so calming.

When something bad has occurred with a patient and stress is mounting, I find the following exercise beneficial: when I can objectively remember that my patient selection, my technical and thoughtful delivering of care, and my patient interactions were all in order, it brings me peace. When I know there's nothing that I would have done differently or will do differently in the future, this realization goes a long way in fighting fear and anxiety. Such self-coaching can be very assuring. And in other situations in which you realize that you should have done things differently, turn that event into a positive learning opportunity.

Unfortunately, there's only one way to guarantee having no complications, no untoward outcomes, and no unhappy patients: by not practicing medicine. But for the sake of your patients, and the sake of yourself, you cannot give up.

Be Proud of Yourself

When you have shouldered a fearful, complicated, or stressful situation, be proud of yourself. Pride knows when you've done well. It knows when you've kept your composure and chose to react positively in difficult conditions. Pride encourages, brings joy, and is an endless source of fist pump opportunities.

Though often fleeting, it affirms and promotes gratitude. And before you know it, stress and fear are replaced by healthier thoughts and more fulfillment.

Learn from Others

Many physicians learn successful mental battle strategies from other professionals. Highly skilled life coaches and psychologists are readily available, as are numerous books and teaching apps. Resilience training and meditation are commonly used to manage stress and reduce burnout.

Some Practical Legal Maneuvers

In addition to mental battle strategies, I suggest that you take a number of practical maneuvers that may prove beneficial in reducing stress around the culture of litigation.

Document, Document, Document

I have an inherent bias for keeping detailed medical records, and heartily recommend good documentation, especially if you sense any impending trouble or issues with any patient. Proactively document if a patient's behavior appears odd or out of context, or if his or her expectations are alarmingly unrealistic. Sometimes just a gentle red flag sensitizing your antennas to future encounters may be beneficial. Your sixth sense of being cautious can be very valuable.

Document when and why the patient is unhappy, angry, if they haven't reached their treatment goal, and any other instances. Rude or inappropriate remarks and behavior to you or your staff should be noted as well. Don't be afraid to include a detailed representation of words spoken both by you and by the patient.

When a patient is out of line, I place their words almost verbatim into the medical record. When I'm firm and abrupt, it's documented, including the fact that I was simultaneously polite and professional. Recognizing the patient has a full right to their medical record or may view it online, I don't hesitate to dictate the truth.

It's amazing how when a patient complains to administration, your staff, or in rare cases to the medical board or an attorney, the facts of the case and truth of the encounter often change. More bluntly, it can be shocking how grossly many will lie, vindictively seeking revenge or restitution. Most commonly it's about money, poor outcomes, or complications that the patient is unwilling to accept.

But remember, it greatly reduces stress and strengthens your case and resolve when proactive and transparent documentation already exists in their medical record. Document, document, document. The threat of the much too common "he said she said" is minimized.

Practice Literature-Based Medicine
Practicing literature-based medicine with a strong bias toward first using conservative therapies reduces stress associated with our litigation culture. I think it's easier to defend when litigated, and it gives both the provider and patient more peace of mind and less apprehension when less invasive therapies were exhausted first.

It was ingrained in me as a trainee and now as a surgeon to always play the devil's advocate when recommending surgery. I stress why a patient may not reach their treatment goal or be satisfied with their results. I highlight any patient-specific increased concerns for a noted complication or outcome, and all are highlighted in my preoperative discussion and documentation. I think this approach is more protective as it pertains to litigation.

In contrast, I've always wondered how surgeons who appear to have pretty liberal indications for recommending surgery deal with the stress when patients are unhappy due to poor outcomes. Depending on your level of agreeableness, unhappy patients will ruin your day. If such stress is weighing you down, if you are an aggressive surgeon or provider, perhaps taking a second look at your therapeutic approach might be beneficial.

It's All About Communication

The patient-physician relationship is healthier when communication between both parties is honest, transparent, and proactive. Under the philosophy that the truth always wins, such an approach reduces stress, fear, and associated burnout.

If you are concerned that you may not be able to reach the patient's treatment goal, *tell them*. If some aspects of their tests, procedure, or treatment did not go fully as planned, they need to know. It's not your fault that their tissues were already scarred, their body habitus made the surgery more difficult, that the biopsy did not hit the bullseye as anticipated. Be transparent and proactive with your communication. Patients don't want to learn of these issues in the rearview mirror.

It's best practice to call a patient the day following surgery or invasive procedure to check on their progress. Unlike prescribing a pill, invasive therapies are more likely to have problems that adversely affect care and patient satisfaction.

If a problem exists, deal with it immediately by phone or in person. If a patient is sick, angry, or concerned, they usually want to see their physician as soon as possible and not an APP. Hiding from disgruntled patients will only disgruntle them further.

Empathy, caring, and identifying with the patient's issue and their perception of the problem is important. Many times, their anger and finger-pointing can be quickly diffused by a listening ear and comforting words. They want to be heard. They want to be helped. They want things to be taken care of. Not surprisingly, many are frightened.

Having said that, when appropriate, don't be afraid to be honest with the patient. Don't hesitate to politely reset the facts and the decision process that was made. Summarize the case, your recommendations, their treatment decisions. Remind them of your role in helping them as their physician. Blending empathy and professionalism, it's important to set the record straight and document it.

Don't allow the old switcheroo to rule the day. Nip it in the bud. The old switcheroo will repaint and reset the facts of the case forever and you'll be sacrificed. In a world of blaming others and loss of civility, physicians need to stand up for themselves. We don't exist to take on others' responsibility and to be victimized. Remember: the truth wins.

Don't Get in Trouble Alone

Especially for surgeons and those performing invasive procedures, I recommend that you follow the golden rule: when you anticipate trouble or you're experiencing a significant complication, don't get in trouble alone.

Call for reinforcements. It's no time to be prideful. Even when you think you can effectively manage a situation, don't hesitate to ask a partner or colleague for a fresh set of hands or eyes. Second opinions for any difficult issue or decision drive excellence, reduce stress, and documentation of this can be very beneficial. As is the case with Stephen the general surgeon, a team approach improves care and reduces stress and burnout.

If the Worst Happens, Call the Experts

I feel awful when an angry patient is advancing their complaint toward actionable steps and even litigation. There's that knot in the gut, slumped shoulders, a sudden cold sweat; for moments it's nearly impossible to concentrate. In the midst of trying to help others, it's such a stress-provoking and fearful experience.

As noted with any acute stressor, first narrow your concentration to the daily tasks at hand, and then deal with the problem as soon as you're able. Most important, seek help from the experts. Don't call the patient. Don't discuss potential litigation issues with staff and others. Call the experts.

Our administrator is excellent when dealing with these circumstances. Armed with the knowledge of the patient-physician relationship, the importance of the issue to me, my group, and the regulatory boards, he takes over the problem. He understands the importance of hearing from all sides, especially the unhappy patient. He effectively handles all the sharp edges in an attempt to resolve a stressful and sensitive issue.

Our attorneys and insurance carrier are immediately notified for their awareness and consultation. The weight lifted off one's burdened shoulders knowing that experts are effectively managing the situation is calming and relieving.

Team Talk

Navigating the environment of litigation is challenging for nurses and APPs. Here are a few suggestions to help you adapt and to be successful.

Be Your Best

All providers benefit from being their best while caring for patients. Consistently bringing your A game will help protect you from outside criticism as well as grant you confidence and calm.

Self-analysis of what you do well and what knowledge and skills you need to develop is important. Healthcare is rapidly changing and regular updating of skills is necessary. Use the world of information and available resources in the community, and don't be afraid to ask a colleague for instruction or help. "There is never a dumb question" applies to all.

Diffuse and Document

Nurses commonly speak with patients who are upset, complaining, and critical of the care they have received. These interactions are increasing and stressful to providers.

Learning how to diffuse such a situation is beneficial. For some it comes naturally, and for others the skill can be learned. Identifying and empathizing with the patient's concern is vital. Diligent follow-up is always appreciated. Focus your energy on the patient's expectations, but have boundaries, and do what is reasonable and within your control.

It's important to protect yourself by gently reminding patients that you are trying to help and that you would appreciate being spoken to appropriately. Document untoward interactions and be specific and thorough with your account. Don't be afraid to document the truth. The truth may turn out to be your best friend just when you need it.

Remember the Lifelines

Like physicians, nurses and APPs regularly feel overwhelmed and in need of a lifeline. Compartmentalizing and checking off one task at a time is a lifeline for many. Also, medicine is a team sport. Ask for help or freely offer a helping hand to someone in distress. An outstretched arm is a lifeline that flows in both directions.

A JOURNEY MOMENT

If you are battling burnout and fear, it's important to identify the enemy. For instance, is it your technical skills, your confidence, adverse outcomes and sequelae, an unhappy customer, failure, or other? List what you are fearful of or concerned about.

_____

_____

_____

_____

_____

_____

_____

_____

Are the issues actually true, or are they somewhat perceived or emotionally based? Take your time and really think about them. Write down your thoughts—it's important to be transparent and truthful.

_____

_____

_____

_____

_____

_____

_____

Look for strategies in this chapter that might be helpful. Apply them specifically to you and set up a game plan to incorporate them into your thoughts and life. Don't be afraid to discuss your fears with a colleague, a best friend, or spouse. Their objective and comforting words may be life-giving.

Chapter 20

Big Pharma and Burnout

Possibly the biggest target of criticism for the skyrocketing cost of healthcare is directed toward the pharmaceutical industry and those who fall somewhat more under the radar—the manufacturers of medical devices and equipment. Headline after headline, TV pundits, and maybe even you and your best friend blame the pharmaceutical industry for the high cost of healthcare. There's no question that for many, Big Pharma is the bad guy.

Before continuing, I need to be transparent about my relationship with the makers of drugs and equipment, as it could be viewed as making me biased.

I serve on the senior physician advisory board of multiple companies that produce medications and products in my therapeutic space. As a key opinion leader and subsequent advisor, I participate in early phase study design, in the interpretation and publication of data, and the dissemination of that data through publications, academic meetings, and by lecturing to colleagues and other physicians.

The financial reimbursement associated with some of these activities is highly regulated and scrutinized by the FDA. The amounts I've received are often in the tens of thousands of dollars annually. I've had these relationships for decades.

I have mixed feelings when it comes to the greed virus and how it's infected manufacturers of drugs and equipment. Behind the scenes, I've regularly witnessed a genuine attempt by the industry to make products that help physicians achieve excellence and better treat their patients. I've witnessed the entrepreneurial spirit of America in the development of world-class products that help millions. With the rarest of exceptions, I've not seen sleaziness or dishonesty; their level of professionalism is noteworthy. I'm proud of my relationship with the industry and it's been an honor to be professionally associated with them.

Having said that, I agree that many of the pharmaceutical products are brutally expensive and arguably not affordable to patients and our healthcare system. Like the insurance industry, the makers of drugs and equipment are in the business of making money, and guess what? They've succeeded. They are printing money and our country is paying for it.

In 2016, the total revenue of the global pharmaceutical market was estimated to be $1.05 trillion, with a *t*, boasting very high profit margins. Putting that into perspective, it's roughly one-quarter of what the U.S. federal government spends annually. And more than 50 percent of their revenue is made here in the U.S. and Canada.

The Great Debate on Profits

Let's take a few moments and debate whether you're for or against Big Pharma and other manufacturers and their high profitability. Because whether you like it or not, there are two sides to the story.

"You can't have your cake and eat it too" is a popular figure of speech, one I was accustomed to hearing regularly growing up in eastern Canada. Once the cake is eaten, it's gone. The proverb's meaning is similar to the phrases "you can't have it both ways," and "you can't have the best of both worlds."

For those against Big Pharma, paying $400 a month for a drug is unacceptable, especially for common and benign conditions. New cancer drugs costing tens of thousands annually while prolonging life by only a few months are inappropriate. It is wrong that hospital device representatives selling hip prosthesis and pacemakers enjoy incomes that often surpass the surgeons that are actually doing the surgery. If the rep can be paid so handsomely, how much is the profit?

All these costs and profits are driving up insurance premiums and threatening the financial solvency of Medicare. They're threatening the financial health of individuals, businesses, and our nation.

You can guarantee that these prices will continue to increase, ensuring multi-million-dollar CEO compensation, their reward for increasing the company's Wall Street value. **Like all publicly owned businesses, it's all about the stock price—the ticker tape drives the endless greed virus. But corporate greed and its enormous profit is not sustainable.**

On the other side of the argument, if pharmaceutical companies can't generate annual revenues in the several hundreds of millions from a new medication, they'll not risk the vast amount of money that went into the research and development of the drug. Based on patent life, they only have a limited number of years to recoup their investment.

Society will no longer benefit from new treatments for everyday health conditions like migraine headaches and hypertension. The next big therapeutic breakthrough for diabetes or stroke may not happen. If corporations cannot drive profits high enough to keep their investors happy, prostate cancer will have fewer treatment options if it spreads. Current therapies for metastatic prostate cancer are helping millions, and they're helping millions because they make money.

Already Big Pharma is steering away from developing medications that have competing products, especially generics, because profits are lower. Even if the new drug is superior, third-party payers regularly refuse coverage and demand the use of generics, even if they're less effective. In response, Big Pharma has directed much of its research and development toward highly priced oncology drugs and to treating conditions in which new therapies are more difficult to deny coverage.

I'm currently working with a company that hopes to significantly impact the treatment of urinary incontinence by bringing to market a new office-based procedure. This company would have never been able to raise the necessary investor capital for its research and development unless the device eventually is highly profitable, and yes, that means expensive.

Although at face value it appears harsh, you could make the following argument to those against Big Pharma: if you don't like the price of a therapy, then simply live without it. No one's forcing you to be treated and we do live in a capitalistic society.

Consider this: you would be living without the therapy since the company wouldn't have developed it in the first place. And that would adversely affect the care of millions of others who are willing to pay. Simply put, you can't have your cake and eat it too.

But What About Lower-Priced Meds in Canada?

The most avid criticizers of Big Pharma and others regularly tout how much lower the price for drugs is in Canada. Drive across the border and it's half price. That's often used as a talking point demanding lower prices.

The reason for this is that Canada limits access of drugs and equipment into the country unless the industry significantly reduces its pricing. For them, their take-it-or-leave-it approach has generally fared them well, but in some cases, treatments north of the border aren't available as a result.

What critics fail to mention (purposely or not), is that if the U.S. flexed the same posture, many of the products wouldn't ever be developed. It's that simple. It's the highly profitable U.S. market that pays for American research and development and the rest of the world benefits from the discounts. Yes, America is the inventor for the rest of the world.

Setting the Record Straight About Physician Relationships with Pharma

I'm proud of my consulting relationship with the pharmaceutical industry. It's enabled me to contribute to my subspecialty advancing patient care and excellence. But there's no question that such relationships have been abused by some, sometimes grossly so, and many cases are in the public domain.

But to set the record straight, the financial relationship between physicians and industry is not increasing the cost of drugs and equipment. The budget allotted for this is a fraction of the company's overall operating expenses.

Instead, the price of drugs and equipment is driven by the cost that the market will bear, and up until now, that number has been very high. To say that the price of that little blue pill enhancing erections was $20 because a physician was reimbursed for giving an industry-sponsored educational talk is simply untrue and naïve.

Similarly, to say that physicians prescribe medication because the industry buys them lunch is laughable and insulting.

What's really escalating prices year after year is the greed virus infecting the industry and its insatiable need to drive up stock value. It's why a company worth billions wants more. And like insurance companies, their lobbyists are influencing politicians and this goes all the way to the White House.

Remember, when it comes to healthcare, you and I are living on Main Street, and we now exist for a whole bunch of people to make a whole bunch of money. And regardless of corporate speak and mission statements, in many cases altruism is not the industry's primary directive.

What About the Free Market?

Capitalists argue that the forces of supply and demand and the free market in healthcare will successfully dictate prices and value.

I disagree.

The greed virus infecting manufacturers of drugs and equipment has driven the cost of their products and subsequently healthcare through the roof, independent of how much the consumer and system are able to afford. The forces of the free market are not working; unchecked prices continue to rise. Without regulations, the train of higher prices and profit has already left the station and is only going to travel faster.

My hope is that Big Pharma and others will someday realize that even they can't have their cake and eat it too. Their capitalistic pricing is threatening the financial health of individuals and our nation. Something's got to give. It's not sustainable.

Costs of Pharma and the Relationship with Burnout

In the case of manufacturers of drugs and equipment and how they relate to physician burnout, my thoughts are limited. Being their customer, industry benefits when they have a good relationship with us, especially in a competitive marketplace.

During a stressful day, a visit by a pharmaceutical representative may be annoying, but it doesn't have any long-term effects and the short-term consequences are relatively miniscule. The annoyance is not their fault, but usually from them showing up and messaging about their product at the wrong time. Our practice has an open-door policy regarding representatives, but we try to limit our exposure to planned times or during lunch.

The high price of products and equipment adds increasing financial pressure to private practices, especially in the midst of lower reimbursements. The cost of electronic medical records, lasers, ultrasound machines, and supplies continues to rise, while third-party payers pay us less. The resulting profit margin of many office-based procedures like biopsies and endoscopy is ridiculous. Many practices with high volumes have benefitted from negotiating lower pricing with vendors. It's sometimes necessary for physicians to perform poorly reimbursed procedures in the hospital to prevent losses.

When patients are financially stressed, there often comes with it a loss of civility. In our office, we regularly bear the brunt of a patient's unpleasantness who is grappling with high costs. Patients endlessly complain about not being able to afford medications, and too often we as physicians are blamed for this. Balancing empathy with healthy boundaries is a good strategy in these circumstances.

When patient care suffers as a result of economics, we all are frustrated. Remaining focused on delivering excellence will motivate and sustain you.

I believe one of the knock-on effects of higher pharmaceutical costs and equipment is that Medicare lowers its physician reimbursement as their easiest target in their attempts to reduce government spending. Politicians know that physicians are getting financially creamed, and they don't care. Big Pharma, their lobbyists, and government win. Physicians and patients lose. As the cost of doing business increases for traditional insurance companies, they too sacrifice physician reimbursement in their attempts to lower premiums and enrich profit.

But in general, the presence of the pharmaceutical and medical products industry in the daily lives of physicians is positive and resourceful. Their greed virus affecting physician burnout is minimal. They smile, they thank us, they're respectful, they educate providers about their products. And enjoying a hot lunch from time to time is okay too. On behalf of all physicians, I thank Big Pharma and others for their support and assistance.

Pharma: We Need Your Help
Let's face it, academic meetings and medical education websites arguably wouldn't exist without the makers of drugs and equipment underwriting the expenses associated. Without sponsorship, continuing medical education would be severely impacted.

Recognizing the educational value that these companies bring to the healthcare industry, they could also be an ally in our battle against burnout. As part of my mission to lift up physicians and those who serve, I'm dedicating time and energy to inspiring the makers of drugs and equipment to join us as partners in this endeavor.

Big Pharma and medical device companies should sponsor awareness and education about physician burnout. I encourage them to bring us resources and experts benefitting all. Just talking about burnout could be life-changing to many.

Apathy, loss of joy, burnout—all are enemies to delivering excellence to patients. Enemies to the health of our nation. The benefit of lifting up physicians and providers would be compounding and generational. And more excellence would financially benefit Big Pharma and others.

So, to Urovant, to Astellas, to Valencia, to Medtronic, to all of our wonderful corporate partners, speaking for physicians, for patients, and for our nation, we need your help.

We need your help by continuing to bring us wonderful new treatments enabling us to provide excellence.

We need your help in reducing healthcare costs. The endless rising cost of medications and equipment is not sustainable. The day that you cannot have your cake and eat it too is rapidly approaching.

And importantly, we need your help in our battle against burnout. Please help bring us the resources, the education, and the experts to help us find joy and fulfillment providing care for our nation.

TEAM TALK

The endless pre-authorizations needed for expensive medications is frustrating and discouraging, but whether to blame Big Pharma or third-party payers is debatable.

Work with your pharmaceutical representative who can provide you tips and tricks to get medications more easily approved. Record your notes in your "bible of excellence" binder. Use the co-pay cards and samples. Ask your physician to provide you with talk tracks that will help you expedite the process. And enjoy the representative's hot lunch or a few snacks. You never know when a friendship will kindle.

A Journey Moment

Do you think that the greed virus infecting the makers of drugs and equipment adversely affects your burnout? If yes, provide at least two examples and include any action(s) that you can take to reduce your stress.

1. _____
   _____
   _____
   _____
   _____
   _____
   _____
   _____

2. _____
   _____
   _____
   _____
   _____
   _____
   _____

CHAPTER 21

THE HOSPITAL GREED VIRUS: THE COMMODITIZATION OF HEALTHCARE

One of the greatest changes to healthcare in the last two decades has been the corporatization of our hospitals into multi-billion-dollar healthcare systems, and the indoctrination of the culture of Wall Street into our hospitals.

Like so many other industries, healthcare systems continue to expand in their attempts to reduce competition, to survive in difficult markets, and to maximize profit and bargaining power. Whether you like it or not, the business of healthcare and massive healthcare systems are here to stay.

As with any significant transformation, there are going to be pros and cons, winners and losers. Large hospital campuses now provide access, services, and employment arguably far greater than what could have ever been achieved by the original hospital model. But that's come with costs.

Such corporatization did not occur for altruistic or community service reasons, it was done to make money. Healthcare systems and their naturally associated greed virus have significantly increased the costs of healthcare, and in many cases threatened its quality. There's no question that the change in the culture has adversely affected providers, promoting physician stress and burnout.

These healthcare systems function with a similar mindset as any other large business. There's a lot of money that can be made looking after the health needs of the customer named "Patient." But when an individual and their healthcare is assigned too much economic value, then the "market value" of a person can replace the other societal values of humans—and this is where the greed virus train has clearly left the station, perhaps sadly forever.

The Rise of Mega-Hospitals

Having lived and practiced medicine in the United States, Canada, New Zealand, and England, it's fair to say that the majority of the finest hospitals in the world are here in the U.S. Their size, infrastructure, the brain power and expertise that lies within, are a true testimony to capitalism, innovation, and excellence.

These hospitals focus on delivering excellent and safe patient care, and are often the largest and most important employers in their community. Their presence should be truly appreciated.

Mega-hospitals improve profit by cutting costs, in economies of scale, better purchasing power, and stronger negotiating strength, ensuring higher reimbursement from third-party payers and government. Competitiveness is reduced by hospitals owning most of the physicians and other providers, their patients, and arguably, the politicians they lobby.

Their CEOs are reimbursed handsomely. Highly skilled, they navigate endless moving parts and pressure from the lower reimbursement from insurers, the escalating costs of operation, and emergency departments full of the sick and uninsured. With thin profit margins, the hospital environment is tough and not for the faint of heart.

But in spite of such pressure and challenges, successfully run hospitals are tremendously profitable. They seemingly have an unlimited "if you build it, they will come" potential as our society ages, gets sicker, and wants more and more. Just think how fast healthcare systems have expanded, building new oncology centers and surgical suites even during the last major recession when many businesses were failing.

Similar to banks on Wall Street, most large healthcare systems are simply too big to fail. The community's medical and financial health is dependent on the hospital's viability, and trust me, the CEOs running them know it. Their lobbyists influence the local politicians who will do anything to ensure the financial stability of their community's major employer.

So, What's the Problem with Giant Hospitals?

In general, when corporations in an industry expand and take over the landscape, they do so to maximize profit, but unfortunately the profit is rarely shared with the customer or end-user, nor does it lower the cost to the system. In many cases, the corporation gets richer while the end-user and system pay more and receive less.

In the case of healthcare, such corporatization has grossly increased overall costs, adversely affected quality, and promoted physician burnout. The bottom line is that Main Street healthcare is suffering while the hospitals who operate like Wall Street are benefitting greatly.

Functional Monopolies

Healthcare systems in many cases are functional monopolies in their respective local markets. Their instinctive business behavior has driven up costs by multiple means, some of which include pricing power, turbo-charging access, and controlling the kingdom.

Pricing Power

Healthcare systems now employ the majority of physicians, many of whom were struggling to survive as small business owners. The American Medical Association released a survey in May of 2021 showing that the overall number of physicians in wholly physician-owned practices dipped to 49 percent, a 5 point drop from 2018. And the trend is continuing. This reality should bring us pause.

When hospitals employ physicians, the hospitals are reimbursed at much higher rates by Medicare and third-party payers for the same services. This allowance was originally designed to compensate them for providing for the uninsured and for twenty-four-hour care, and the higher compensation referred to as the "facility fee" is substantial.

The powers that be never imagined that hospitals would one day "own" most doctors and now charge a facility fee for the majority of outpatient and office-based visits, lab tests, imaging studies, and procedures. It was estimated that a 49 percent increase in hospital-employed physicians between 2012 and 2015 led to a $3.1 billion increase in Medicare costs related to just four commonly performed procedures, costing patients an additional $400 million. I think that's shameful.

Similarly, healthcare systems owning the majority of patients and providers continually demand higher reimbursement from major insurance providers. A CT scan in a privately-owned physician office might be reimbursed by private insurance for $350, while the same scan in a hospital emergency room or hospital-owned clinic could be over $1,000.

Simply put, hospital pricing power is a scam. Just think about how these gross increases in medical costs are being paid for by your premiums and deductibles, your taxes, and how they're threatening the solvency of Medicare. And at the same time, your politicians, who are fully aware of the fleecing, tout that they care about the cost of healthcare. The same politicians who were responsible for the financial gutting of the private practice physician by Medicaid and Medicare.

Turbo-Charging Access

In addition to pricing power, hospitals have dramatically driven up costs by commoditizing medicine in the minds of the consumer. Like Starbucks, they've turbo-charged access by building massive healthcare campuses, including emergency rooms and urgent care centers, on seemingly every corner.

Patients with headaches and sore stomachs, lured by "10-minute emergency room wait" signs are evaluated with thousands of dollars' worth of tests, when what they really needed was a good night's sleep, a few Tylenol, and some old-fashioned time that cures most aches and pains.

Many urgent care centers are staffed by advanced practice providers and not the more expensive doctors, and exist as profit centers, handing out tests and medications like Frappuccinos. They are absolutely designed to be the tip of the iceberg delivering an endless number of highly profitable patients to the healthcare system as it expands its regional footprint and control. Healthcare systems have been masters at feeding our "I want everything now" culture and believe me, they're just getting started.

Controlling the Kingdom

As healthcare systems expand, they control the kingdom by wisely tailoring their expansion not only to provide services, but to maximize profit. Such expansion and its associated marketing dictates the marketplace by directing patients to more lucrative services.

If women's health and hip surgery pay handsomely, they'll build a women's hospital and an orthopedic surgical center. If neurosurgery pays, they turn less profitable hospital wards into a neurosurgical institute. Poorly reimbursed services, like psychiatric care, by contrast, see resources limited on purpose. The mentally ill are underserved in this country as the greed virus of "not-for-profit" multi-billion-dollar healthcare systems spreads and multiplies.

Pricing power, turbo-charging access, controlling the kingdom. All are accepted as business as usual in a capitalistic society. And sadly, they are printing money as the financial health of individuals, Medicare, and our nation is in jeopardy.

Quality is About the People

I can certainly appreciate pushback regarding my claim that the quality of care has lessened in the hands of these multi-billion-dollar healthcare systems, but I still think I'm right. In spite of these expanding state-of-the-art hospital campuses and "world-class care" signs everywhere, in the greatest country in the world who spends the most on healthcare, quality has actually deteriorated.

Of course, many sectors of hospital-delivered care are phenomenal, but I stand firm in my accusation.

The fundamental problem threatening quality is that the businessmen and their consultants who have taken over healthcare view patients and delivery of care as a business. They see providing healthcare as a tremendous opportunity to make money—that's why they do it. Driving excellence and serving the community is not their primary goal, it's their secondary. And in so many cases, the two goals are in conflict.

In commoditizing the healthcare system, corporate minds applied their instinctive business principles and believe that by using the tools of other industries—like expanding brick-and-mortar infrastructure, improving customer processes, marketing met metrics and customer satisfaction scores, and hiring more administrators—they'll be successful. Arguably correct, their profits have soared, but quality has deteriorated.

Quality has deteriorated because the business model cuts corners for profit and minimizes the value of the people delivering the care. It reduces the importance of the nurses, the ancillary staff, the physicians, and other providers. It sadly minimizes the patient's value and the sanctity of the patient-physician relationship. But when it comes to quality and looking after patients, it's all about the people.

Unlike other industries, in healthcare, the people providing the care are the linchpin in ensuring quality. And sadly, many of the business minds infected with the greed virus have demoted the people to cogs, sacrificing excellence and patient care for profit. With corporate arrogance pervasive, they say, "Move over physicians and other providers, we can do it better."

In spite of beautiful new hospitals with the welcoming valet, smiling greeters, and state-of-the-art equipment, an ever-increasing problem is that a significant number of the providers in healthcare are now less engaged, less knowledgeable, less professional, and too often are not delivering great care.

The Profession of Nursing is Fading

As a supporter of all who serve, it deeply concerns me that the "white cap" days of nursing are fading. Symbolized by the white caps they used to wear, nursing was once a proud profession of excellence and a lifelong calling where one could use gifts and talents to serve others. Nurses were vital members of the healthcare team, amplifying the care delivered by physicians. Nurses were making independent decisions, truly understanding their patients' conditions and their role in caring for them. Willing to go the extra mile, when it came to the patient, the buck stopped with the nurse. Yes, once a proud profession, but now a fading profession that is under siege.

Nursing has become over-corporatized and devalued, and when you mix in changes in the American work ethic, the profession and career of nursing is sadly being replaced by a job with reasonable pay and good benefits. A profession that used to be centered in patient care, nurses are now being forced to sit at computers checking boxes rather than caring for patients. Independent proactive decisions are now a ghost of the past. In fact, independence and a lot of decision-making is deemed outside their scope of practice.

Experience is being replaced by undertrained, less interested, and lower paid staff, frustrating physicians and other nurse colleagues, and adversely affecting patient care.

And sadly, hidden behind their smiles, nursing morale is plummeting. Nurses are increasingly being asked to do more with less, work longer hours, and are not fooled by the corporate talk that "it's all about the patient."

Unfortunately, a caring nurse is often confronted by rude patients and their families, and even by physicians like myself who might be angry for other reasons. They are unable to defend themselves to patients and family members since in the hospital setting the "customer" is always right.

With loyalty no longer valued or fostered, it's commonplace for nurses to jump ship to another job that pays a few extra dollars an hour. Many nurses are burned out and leaving the profession altogether, while others leave hospital nursing to work in less stressful settings like physician offices or outpatient clinics. Many with drive and inspiration join administration or become advanced prectice providers.

Nationwide, patient care is threatened by a shortage of highly qualified nurses in multi-billion-dollar hospital systems. As the nursing profession has become devalued, the supply of excellent nurses has dwindled. Meanwhile, administration and consultants assume little responsibility and chalk it up as a natural part of doing business.

All Providers Are Affected

The corporatized business model that's adversely affecting quality does not stop with nursing.

Advanced practice providers are being hired at astounding rates in an attempt to fill the ever-increasing turbo-charged access. They are taking on more responsibility and being supervised less. APPs play an integral role in delivering care, but when they become under-supervised, quality can be jeopardized, especially in acute settings like the emergency department and intensive care.

Many hospital-employed physicians feel devalued and disrespected as a voiceless provider in the healthcare system. They are frustrated by endless rules and regulations, and discouraged in having to meet reimbursable metrics and keep the patients satisfied. Personal survival and pleasing the administration become the goal, versus providing excellent care.

I'm also concerned that an employed physician "working shifts" may not deliver the same level of care as he or she would in private practice. It's more tempting to shy away from one's duty and responsibility when the patient is perceived as being under the care of the hospital and not the physician. It's also natural for continuity of care to be disrupted when multiple "shift" providers are looking after the same patient.

Many providers are pressured by the hospital to see more and more patients, adversely affecting quality and further promoting physician burnout. It's well established that burnout is associated with medical errors and poor quality of care. The corporate solution seems to be providing yoga classes, a burnout committee, and resilience training for their physicians, but seem unwilling to change the culture or to reduce the workload. Instead, many continue to double down on what's profitable, because although it may take time, the physicians will eventually get with the program.

Community Hospitals Are Dying

The most adversely affected by mega-healthcare systems and their ill effects on providers and quality are small towns and their community hospitals. As was the case with small retail stores and Walmart, the landscape of medicine is too harsh for community hospitals to survive independently, and subsequently they have been absorbed by the system.

Many community hospitals are now functioning as a satellite of the multi-billion-dollar mother ship. The once vibrant, all-purpose community hospital is now unable to recruit and retain good physicians and providers, and so it is increasingly functioning more like an outpatient referral center, but still flies the "world-class care" signs.

Limiting care locally with all arms referring to the centralized campus in the larger city seems like a perfect business paradigm. The CEOs have no interest in duplicating services and paying what it takes to recruit good providers; it's just business.

However, the downside of this plan is that rural Americans are now the biggest losers. As their premiums and deductibles soar, they are regularly driving a few hours to the city with those local hospital "world-class care" signs in their rearview mirror, in order to receive advanced healthcare.

Lack of Trust Promotes Burnout

The people doing the caring in these large hospital systems—the doctors, the nurses, and other providers—are not being cared for. Instead they're being sacrificed for profit, customer service, and a satisfied patient experience. For met metrics and marketing slogans.

The cogs have become a necessary part of doing business, a means to an end. Their personal talent and dreams are relegated to become a faceless employee. As a result, it brings about provider apathy, mediocrity, and an every-man-for-himself mentality. It also looks like lack of excellence, and burnout.

Unfortunately, in many healthcare communities, the providers and hospitals are trying to function together while at odds with one another. Physician and staff turnover is high, and it's difficult to recruit good providers to serve.

The fundamental issue, I believe, is trust. Many physicians and providers don't think that the hospital and its administrators really have their backs. Such a reality cannot be hidden.

A common belief among physicians is that a patient complaint or low satisfaction score, independent of facts and circumstances, is weighed more heavily than our decades of service and honest attempts to treat everyone respectively and to deliver excellence. This reality hurts and discourages the relationship between providers and administration.

There is also a belief among physicians that if hospital profits were threatened, that our compensation would be significantly impacted. That doesn't foster loyalty when one has dedicated their life and career to serving a community that may desperately need their services.

Many of us believe hospitals expanding their campus footprint and actively promoting 24–7 urgent care and emergency room services are sacrificing the health and welfare of their physicians in order to do so. As a physician, I can't continue to work harder, take more call burden, and satisfy the insatiable appetite of consumer healthcare. I'm fatigued, I'm stressed, I'm burning out.

In addition, many providers feel that their goals do not align with those of the hospital, that we don't believe in what they believe. We don't share the same purpose, we don't live the same why. In spite of well-intended mission statements and corporate speak, providing a workplace enabling us to use our gifts and talents to serve and to help others is not the primary goal of most healthcare systems. **Yes, a lack of trust and not believing in the values and mission of the system are strong predictors of physician and provider burnout.**

See, when you operate healthcare like a big-box store, in many cases you get big-box store results: highly functional, highly profitable, but with diminishing quality, and not enough excellence. And unfortunately, unlike the millions of customers enjoying lower prices at Walmart, the patient, the third-party payers, and Medicare are now paying astronomically more for their goods and services.

TEAM TALK

Nurses have been devalued and their morale is plummeting. Many feel like a faceless employee asked to do more with less. The profession has been sacrificed for profit and for customer service. Countless nurses don't share the same vision with their employer or trust who they work for.

Still, the healthcare consultants shamelessly blame COVID-19 as the reason why tens of thousands of nurses have left their jobs. It's an interesting rationalization from the corporate minds that ruined healthcare by making it a commodity. Their greed virus message is a common talk track and influences the groupthink.

The impact of the pandemic and how it has physically and emotionally stressed providers and burned out frontline workers causing them to leave should never be underestimated. But the virus's impact on nurses and the mass exodus represents a much deeper problem.

COVID-19 ripped away the scab that was covering a wound that nurses and advanced practice providers have suffered for more than a decade. It uncovered mistrust, discouragement, frustration, fatigue, voicelessness, and other feelings that providers have toward their employer. And for many, the pandemic represented the last straw. "This is not worth it; I'm out of here," became the new reality.

Without the underlying wound, the fight against COVID-19 could have played out differently. If you don't believe me, just ask the military. When the military is faced with enormous challenges it fights as one and no one leaves the battlefield. They fight with all hands on deck, all believing in the mission. The soldiers and leaders trust one another and are bonded by a brotherhood of love and respect.

Instead, nurses are leaving in droves and many will never return to the job that they once loved. And the quality and delivery of healthcare in the greatest country in the world who spends the most on healthcare is now in jeopardy.

Nice job, consultants, nice job.

A JOURNEY MOMENT

Do you feel like a cog in the wheel of the corporatized healthcare system?

If yes, do you think it adversely affects your joy and fulfillment?

_____

_____

_____

_____

_____

_____

_____

Take a few moments and write down some of your thoughts and feelings regarding this situation. Be honest with yourself. Are you frustrated? Fatigued? Angry? Trying to convince yourself that you don't care? Perhaps saddened or discouraged?

_____

_____

_____

_____

_____

_____

_____

_____

Do you think that your thoughts and feelings are beginning to affect your performance at work? If so, how?

_____

_____

_____

_____

CHAPTER 22

EMBRACING THE CHANGED LANDSCAPE
OF HEALTHCARE SYSTEMS

It's fair to say that the landscape has changed, and multi-billion-dollar health-care systems are here to stay. In fact, the consolidation will likely continue until there are only a few competing players per state or region.

With such a situation, the majority of physicians and providers will forever be employed by these systems, and many others will be dependent on them in order to work and survive. Without a change in corporate culture, a physician becomes a replaceable employee, a shift worker, a means to an end now so common in other industries. And our associated loss of control and autonomy becomes a tremendous source of physician frustration and burnout.

But I believe that physicians can still thrive and be satisfied within this system, and that the profession can be life-giving to providers and those who serve. For those who are fighting burnout or trying to find joy within this changed landscape, they must embrace it in order to be successful in their journey.

Yes, embrace it. Because fighting the changed landscape with conventional tactics and wisdom will not be successful. Look, I want to fight. I want to complain, criticize, and resist when I can. I want to push back and *insist* that the system change. But unfortunately, this is not a winning strategy.

So, the question is: How do physicians find fulfillment when they're employed or dependent on a healthcare system and don't believe in what the hospital believes? When their values and goals don't align with those of the institution? When they don't trust or feel safe in their working environment?

I do not have a magic bullet. I'm still hopeful that my thoughts will be helpful to many of you pursuing your mountaintop amidst a difficult climb to the summit.

So, let's get started. Let me make a few suggestions to help you embrace the landscape and be joyous and fulfilled when Walmart meets healthcare.

The Freedom of Acceptance

Critical to embracing the landscape is acceptance. No matter one's circumstances, finding joy as a healthcare provider really comes down to the decision to take ownership and accept the world of medicine we now live in. Yes, we are employed; yes, we are less valued; yes, multi-billion-dollar healthcare systems are here to stay. But we need to accept it and embrace the changed landscape.

Acceptance and taking personal responsibility will open the door to a new foundation and perspective that will direct your thoughts, emotions, choices, and actions. It can be liberating to you and to those around you.

Acceptance provides you with the freedom to look up. Looking up is where you define and envision your glorious mountaintop, regardless of your circumstances. By looking up, you can make mountaintop decisions, choosing to follow the difficult ascent to the summit. Those physicians refusing to accept the landscape, many with their heads down and shoulders slumped, are no longer climbing.

Battle the thoughts that are dragging you down: your thoughts of the past, your thoughts of how it should be. Battle against your stubborn unaccepting mindset, that too often leads you down into the valley of frustration, bitterness, and resentment. This is a battle I and others fight on a daily basis, and too many of us are losing.

Yes, there is freedom of acceptance, and freedom of looking up. It's so simple, so difficult, but so life-giving.

Taking Personal Responsibility for Your Own Joy

Freed by acceptance, you can then take personal responsibility to ensure your own joy. Relying on others to give you happiness is not likely to be successful.

When taking responsibility, it's important to remember who you are. I believe that the letters *MD* have been engraved into your soul for a reason. That your calling and responsibility weren't randomly chosen, and certainly wasn't granted to be minimized or wasted. It wasn't granted so that you could be mediocre, punch a clock, work a shift, or be burned out and retire early.

Whether you like it or not, the health of the nation rests on your shoulders, and your responsibility as a healer is a heavy cross to bear. You have a life-giving purpose bestowed only to a few, so please don't waste it.

I sometimes wonder if having a heavy cross to bear is part of the journey; in fact it may be what makes the journey an especially meaningful one. That to those given so much responsibility and purpose, there comes a price. And the greater the responsibility and purpose, the greater the weight placed on one's shoulders. The steeper is one's climb to their mountaintop. The heavier their cross.

As is the case with so many trials and tribulations, the struggle is what makes the journey valuable. It is what makes our mountaintop gratifying, having experienced the battles we fought to live out our purpose. Some battles we might win, others are lost. But at the end, we can proudly stand on our summit proclaiming, "Job well done." We finished strong.

Like the Olympian gripping gold as their country's flag is lifted. Like the world-class violinist who gave their life to their art, the Vietnam veteran who fought to keep his brothers safe, the parent of six successful children. Like Jesus carrying a cross through the streets of Jerusalem to his crucifixion, willingly accepting his anointed purpose. All of our life's commitments are all crosses to bear. To those who endure and lift up and carry their heavy cross, all are blessed with fulfillment. Pick up your cross, my friend. Take responsibility and remember who you are.

Lead from Within

Next to a nice dinner and spending time with my family, there's probably nothing I enjoy more than my regular ninety-minute massage with Lori, my friend and masseuse for more than a decade.

In between moans and groans, trigger points melting away from my right gluteal still in spasm, we both laughed loudly on a recent visit. I'd spoken to her regarding what I'm writing about leadership, and Lori uttered, "That's too hard, I think it's easier just to go home and be miserable." I'm still giggling because she might be right.

With acceptance and taking personal responsibility, you can take action and embrace the landscape by leading from within. You can become a leader within a giant organization. You are a source of meaning for yourself, and more importantly, for those around you.

A leader is one who lifts up and helps those next to them, building caring and loving relationships with others. It's asking your staff how their weekend was, and actually listening to the answer. It's asking them for their input regarding patient care, asking about their concerns and frustrations, and empowering them to make decisions and feel safe to fail. Empowerment is such a wonderful gift. Trust is priceless.

Lead from within and build a small team of like-minded persons who share the same purpose, the same why, the same beliefs as healthcare providers. Who share a common lofty vision and goal. Build a team of people who are crying out to feel like they are a part of something special, where they can feel safe and trust one another. Then, gradually but intentionally, expand your circle of friends and influence and incorporate others.

Start with a floor nurse, a secretary, a partner, or better still, an administrator. You'll know the right one. Identify your target. Be proactive. Be a leader and take action.

Your words and actions can be so powerful, and your outreached hand can rescue a soul. Listening and caring in the midst of chaos could help change someone's path forever. Don't underestimate your strength as a physician to lead others—so many look up to that suit of armor.

With time and consistent caring and respect, wonderful and meaningful relationships will develop. Bonded by safety and trust, loyalty and joy will be cultivated, all a result of you leading from within. The power of compounding incremental love and respect will benefit so many.

Lifting up others is not easy, especially when you're struggling yourself. On too many days I agree with Lori that it seems easier just to go home and wallow in my misery. But I want to remind you of your purpose. I want to remind you that you're the best of the best. That you can succeed, adapt, and persist when others can't.

Physicians are the Marines of the corporate work force. I suggest this as your motto: *I refuse to lose. I refuse to be burned out, not joyful, and not fulfilled. I did not come this far and give my life to the profession of medicine to be defeated by corporatized healthcare. I will use my gifts, my talents, and so importantly, my compassion and determination to lead from within and to help others around me.*

Lighten Your Pack

In order to embrace the landscape and to climb to your mountaintop as an employed physician or one who is highly dependent of the healthcare system, you must once again lighten your pack that's weighing you down, slowing your progress, and making you weary.

Too many of us are carrying a pack that is weighed heavily by pride, arrogance, stubbornness, or our unwillingness to yield. It might contain thoughts and words of, "I'm better than you," "You're incompetent," or "You have no clue about how to look after patients."

Let's face it, when it comes to our relationship with hospitals and administrators (that means our bosses), many physicians are pretty lousy employees. Yes, we excel in excellence and conscientiousness, but too often our attitudes and words that we speak are less than acceptable. We would deem that speech unacceptable if the same words were coming from our own employees. In other industries, outward disrespect of the corporate hierarchy is not tolerated. I'm guilty as charged in this respect, but I'm getting better. Many of us still have plenty of work to do.

Of course, physicians are better at patient care and are the masters of the patient-physician relationship versus administrators. So are Lebron and Shack better on the court than their coaches and head office. But if you think that you're an expert in running a hospital—a multi-billion-dollar healthcare system employing thousands of people—get over yourself! You're likely wrong.

I encourage you to lighten your pack and lead from within. Reach out to your administrators, even the ones you perhaps dislike or respect less. The healthcare system and leadership I work with try hard to support its providers and are open to listening to new ideas. Find common ground in attaining mutual goals and objectives. Respect differences in both style and agendas. Learn from one another—everyone has so much to share. A clearer understanding of their side of the story will give you a healthier perspective. Build a synergistic, fruitful relationship. Be transparent. Be malleable. Give a little, take a little. Remember, you're not the only person burdened and pressured by corporate America and life's stresses. And reaching out a hand of care and humility can build some very surprising and amazing relationships.

Remember to be Grateful

Seth, a good friend of mine and fellow urologist, recently fractured the two bones in his lower leg while clearing a lot of land that he was preparing to sell. Seth is employed by his community hospital, and he and his partners bring urologic excellence to Hot Springs, Arkansas.

As an always-smiling and kind-hearted alpha male, Seth sometimes struggled with being employed by others. When he is frustrated, he doesn't mind knocking heads with supervisors and administration. Now injured and with time to reflect, Seth realized some of the benefits of employment. Being gone for many weeks with an almost career-ending injury, he appreciated his modest but adequate compensation while out on leave. If he'd been in private practice with a high overhead, this injury would have been much more financially stressful.

I think too often physicians take for granted many of the benefits associated with being an employed provider.

Generally speaking, employed physicians enjoy a higher income than those in private practice. They are sheltered from changes in reimbursement, from increases in overhead, and are paid the same, regardless of the patient's insurance status. They often work in beautiful new clinics that otherwise might not be affordable. They no longer endure the headaches and responsibility associated with being a small business owner. Remember to be grateful for these wonderful advantages.

Working for a healthcare system opens the door to part-time employment. This can be beneficial to those wishing to slow down later in their career, or when family commitments are more important. Slowing down is difficult in private practice when you are responsible for your full share of the fixed expenses. The margin provided by working part time could also be the solution to those battling with burnout.

Just by simple reframing, your new hospital job can be viewed as a lifeline that rescued you from the woes of private practice. As healthcare systems expand and turbo-charge their access, they are further increasing the relative shortages of physicians. And these shortages help protect us in our relationship with them. It helps protect our lifeline.

Team Talk

The message presented easily applies to all providers. Just think how fortunate you are to have a secure job that enables you to use your gifts to help others.

Lead from within. Your words and actions can be so encouraging to your teammates and you will be blessed for doing so.

A Journey Moment

Leading From Within—An Actionable Step

Identify a person at work with whom you would like to build a trusting relationship. One that will expand your circle of friends and influence. A relationship that will be joyful to all parties.

Cast aside the rushing and chaos and take action. Be brave, be intentional. Speak to them and know that it takes time to build a relationship. Get to know them as a person. Resist gossiping and complaining about work. Listen more, speak less. And when the opportunity arises, reach out a helping hand of trust, safety, and empowerment. Make it about them and not about you. Reap the reward of helping another. Reap the reward of being a leader from within.

And then do it again. Reach out to a staff member, an administrator, or to one of your partners. A brotherhood is built one person at a time. It takes patience to build your circle of friends, your circle of influence. But the significance and joy experienced will benefit all and live forever.

As part of this exercise, write down the names of at least three people that you will reach out to in the next several months. Good luck.

1. _____

2. _____

3. _____

Chapter 23

Be a Voice in Politics

You can make a pretty strong argument that the greatest devastation to our healthcare system and nation has occurred as a result of our greed-infected government and politicians.

I've lived in the U.S. now for nearly three decades, but it still brings me pause when I think about how dishonest many of our politicians are—yes, even the ones I voted for. They truly are an interesting breed: narcissistic, charismatic, and some of them lie so easily. Many make secretive deals, prioritize winning at all costs, and manipulate the public, pretending that they are acting on behalf of their constituents. Somehow, many have become multi-millionaires while making modest salaries, but none have the character to admit how.

Is the Government Really Serving the People?

I'm not sure about you, but I'm often annoyed by a congressman or senator justifying their position by saying that they are "here to serve the American people." That they are in the "people's house doing the people's business." The more and more it's not reality, the more and more they project it as their guiding star, a common defense mechanism of a dishonest ego. Their words are shallow and too often not even close to the truth.

Much of the political class is not here to serve—the political class exists to win. The political class exists for power and control, for money, ego, and to live in a world separate from ours. It exists because partisanship and winning is what's important to a growing number of the public and media who vote for them. And it exists as our society has become increasingly less educated and aware, and more and more dependent on the ruling class. I love America, but Rome is burning.

What's unfortunate about our political environment is what it has done to healthcare. The government has knowingly provided fertile soil for the spread of the greed virus of third-party payers, the makers of drugs and equipment, the hospitals, and litigation attorneys. They have knowingly sacrificed the physician, the nurse, the patient, and the financial health of the nation for their own gain. Remember: when lobbyists win, we lose.

My friend Jeff's healthcare premium is $18,000 annually, with a $7,500 deductible per family member, because the system is rigged by government and third-party payers. The majority of physicians left private practice and joined healthcare systems because the system is rigged by government and hospitals. Frivolous lawsuits and unnecessary regulations will continue to escalate because the system is rigged by government and attorneys. And trust me, the price of drugs and equipment are not going down—the system is rigged.

Let's face it: the financial health of healthcare is failing under the watch of politicians and presidents, all claiming that they are "here to serve." All claiming they care.

It's No Wonder We Suffer from Burnout

The over-corporatization of the healthcare system endorsed by politicians has commoditized our profession and sacrificed physicians' economic and emotional health as a necessary part of doing business. And trust me, our demise is okay with your local congressman and senator.

The government has helped destroy the private practice of medicine when it really didn't need to. One more cut, one more regulation, one more step closer to our failure as a small business. The fall of the profession of medicine as a private practice in the greatest country in the world who spends the most on healthcare will someday be an enlightening historical reflection shining the light on a fallen nation. Shining the light on greed.

The realization of the government greed virus and its relationship with physician burnout can be a difficult pill to swallow. It's difficult to be hopeful when you think that very few of those in power actually care. Recognizing our politicized landscape and that the train has long left the station, I would like to make a few suggestions that might be helpful in fighting against this negative reality.

Be a Voice

It's important for physicians to speak up to our government officials regarding healthcare and burnout. We need to be a voice for ourselves and for others. Speak up, get involved, and take action. Keeping silent and putting our head in the sand is not a good strategy. Pursue the issue that you see as paramount, and don't be afraid of failure. Even going through the process of trying to be heard by your representative may be rewarding.

To be a voice on behalf of physicians can take on many shapes and sizes. Support your medical lobby either financially or with personal time and effort. Our Large Urology Group Practice Association (LUGPA) lobby has been very successful in working with the Centers for Medicare and Medicaid to improve regulatory measures, fee schedules, and to protect ambulatory surgery centers and lithotripsy. I agree with one of the past presidents of LUGPA, noting the importance of advocating for providers: "If we don't fight, we're going to be buried."

But speaking up and lobbying is foreign to many. We lack experience, training, and some feel dirty at just the thought of it, wondering, "Why can't politicians and others just do what's right? Why do we have to fight, or worse, pay for something so obviously good for physicians and healthcare?" But resist stubbornness and living in the past. The days of staying silent and still being successful are over.

Be a voice by voting for like-minded politicians. Vote for those who are more physician-friendly, the ones who actually are concerned for our profession. Better still, run for political office yourself. Get in the waters and swim with the sharks—you never know the greatness you'll achieve. I trust that many physician politicians feel that their efforts in successfully passing beneficial healthcare legislation have been very rewarding versus helping one patient at a time in daily practice.

Be a voice as an employed physician by influencing your hospital to lobby and speak up on behalf of physicians. You're absolutely right that it's not easy. Concentrate your efforts to issues that benefit both you and them. Remember, the hospital lobby is very influential.

Be a voice by unionizing. It's very difficult for physicians to unionize or to go on strike. But you can speak as one through social media. If the medical profession exposed the truths regarding the greed virus of government and corporatized healthcare—in a very professional and truthful way—you would have a headline and change in behavior immediately. Because many in government and corporatized healthcare are spending millions of dollars branding untruths.

It can be hard for physicians to band together, because too often we're focused on our own specialty, or perhaps our own personal set of circumstances. And others know it. We're notorious for just sitting back and taking whatever negative is thrown our way, and our silence points the blame on ourselves as the ultimate problem. M.D. = Make Do. Stop making do. Start making right.

TEAM TALK

Unfortunately, the over-corporatization of the healthcare system endorsed by politicians is here to stay. Nurses and APPs have been sacrificed by the insatiable greed virus of many. The government is making decisions based on politics and macroeconomics benefitting the Wall Street of medicine, and is less interested in the health and well-being of individual providers.

The effects of the pandemic have highlighted that nurses too have a loud and powerful voice to share with others. The nation's critical shortage of them is on the minds of many. The crisis is making national headlines, and trust me—politicians are beginning to hear about it. Even their families and friends sometimes have to go to the emergency room and experience a fifteen-hour wait before being seen.

Nurses have unionized their voice less by speaking, but more so by action. They are speaking with their feet by leaving their job and this has sent a very strong message. "This is not worth it; I'm out of here," is adversely affecting care, but also the pocketbooks of many.

My hope is that the system will wake up and finally hear the voices of nurses and other providers. When given the opportunity, providers should be clear and concise regarding the underlying problem. Higher wages may place a bandage over the wound, but true healing won't occur until the real causes are addressed. It's difficult to put a price tag on feeling appreciated, respected, safe, and knowing that you have a voice that is being heard.

A Journey Moment

Are you discouraged by the greed virus infecting politicians and how it adversely affects you and the profession of medicine?

Can you think of a way you might use your voice to influence government and positively impact physician burnout? Remember, when we band together as one voice, we are much more effective.

_____

_____

_____

_____

_____

_____

_____

_____

_____

_____

CHAPTER 24

PATIENTS OR CUSTOMERS?

A lthough I still continue to struggle with burnout at times, with the strategies I've outlined in this book, I'm so much better than I used to be. It's funny, back when I began writing my book, I had no clue that I was affected, although it may have been obvious to others. Looking back, I realize how writing and exploring ways to battle burnout has been beneficial.

I rarely make angry comments anymore, and my days on the soapbox have almost ceased, thank goodness. I am far less bitter and resentful. Self-awareness is what started me on my current journey on an upward path toward my mountaintop. I can honestly say that for the most part, I'm pretty content being a physician, but three years ago? Heck no! And having recently asked my daughter Lindsey and my wife Andrea about my attitude, they both concur that I was burned out three years ago and am so much happier now.

There's no question that what ticked me off the most about being a physician and what subsequently burned me out was being devalued and disrespected by the system, by others, but most of all, by my patients. Rude, entitled, demanding patients, combined with the pressure of perfection and the culture of litigation can really wear you down. And the commoditization of a once sacred patient-physician relationship now devalued by a satisfaction score is still a difficult pill for me to swallow. Let's face it, the greed and entitlement virus infecting patients is spreading, and I don't think it's good for anyone, especially physicians.

The Patient Care Conundrum

I discuss the greed virus infecting patients because I think many physicians are suffering as a result, even though they may be unaware. Whether it's habit, ego, embarrassment, or what's expected, I think many physicians tout they still like patients and patient care, when in reality they are enormously stressed as a result of looking after them, well beyond the expected and healthy levels of stress associated with practicing medicine. Healthy stress can build one's strength and bring pride and joy. Unhealthy stress can erode the soul.

To win a battle, you first must identify the enemy. To beat stress and burnout, it's imperative to identify and face the demons that are haunting you. If it's the patients and you don't deal with it, you're going to have a difficult climb to your summit of joy, peace, and fulfillment. I believe that one of the turning points for me was the acknowledgment of this reality.

The Four Rs That Will Help You Love Your Patients

I'm embarrassed to admit that in my worst moments, I was actually angry toward some of my patients. Or perhaps better stated, angry toward the American public. Their rudeness, their demands, their entitlement—for me, it was unacceptable. Even patients who were thankful for their surgical care, I would sometimes ponder if they would have turned on me if their surgery had not been successful. I started lumping too many patients into a common sea of ungratefulness: happy when things go their way, and miserable to others when they do not.

Obviously, these thoughts were unhelpful and in the long term, self-destructive.

Let me share with you what I refer to as my four Rs that may be helpful if you're struggling with loving on your patients.

Recognize

The first step in your fight against the patient greed and entitlement virus is for you to *recognize* that it exists. It's no time to sugarcoat it, or pretend it doesn't exist. If the patients are beating you down, it's imperative that you come to terms with that realization.

Having recognized your foe, the next step is to accept. Recognize and accept that some patients will devalue and disrespect you. Recognize and accept that some patients will like or dislike you based on their treatment outcome. Recognize and accept that unfortunately, America has lost some of its civility. This empowers and frees you to look up and choose to follow your upward path to the summit.

Remember

You know the drill. In order to take on the patient greed and entitlement virus you must *remember* your purpose, you must remember your why. Remember that you were given gifts and talents to help others and to serve.

Of course, sacrificing for others is a tough journey. On some days the ascent to your mountaintop may appear impossible. But in these moments of greatest stress and struggle, look up, remember your purpose, be encouraged, and keep on climbing.

Resist

In order to transform wisdom, thoughts, and emotions into positive action, you have to *resist* being in survival mode.

Over time, I found that the system and the patients were wearing me down, and although I remained highly functioning and positive, I inadvertently started going into what I now refer to as survival mode. I adopted a number of actions, but more commonly, *reactions* that I thought protected me in the midst of the perceived chaos. Like in any relationship, when one perpetually feels attacked or betrayed, it's natural in some cases to retaliate.

I became more stern and abrupt with patients who I felt were inappropriate, impossible to please, or complained endlessly. My smiles were rare to those who were not civil. On some occasions I was quick to suggest to patients that they might want to seek care elsewhere if they were not pleased "with our service." At times I was confrontational, arrogant, sometimes almost boastful to my staff regarding my performance, but day after day on my drive home, I was feeling frustrated, agitated, sometimes ashamed, and certainly not joyful and fulfilled.

Looking back, reacting and fighting was a lose-lose interaction. A loss for the patient, a loss for myself and my staff, and too often a loss for my family, who were innocent but exposed to my moods as I brought the battle home. Resist survival mode, resist blame—it's not a good strategy.

Ready

Ready yourself by being proactive. Proactively decide to fight less and smile more. Proactively make a decision to limit survival mode tactics, knowing that empathy and a smile can heal and build bridges, while negative reactions only propagate similar responses in the future. Similarly, the gift of a smile, empathy, and understanding can also be learned, rolling the growing snowball of positivity in the right direction. As we sail through our day, our attitude leaves a wake of energy that will influence, and then reflect off those around us and ultimately return to our own emotional shore. Make those waves as warm and loving as possible.

Be ready by not emotionally distancing yourself too much from patients. This can be a natural response to a dysfunctional intimate relationship, but then the patient-physician relationship becomes robotic, merely a service to a customer, and joy is lost when the patient becomes a commodity. **And worse, when you don't feel close and sympathetic to your patients, you begin to wonder what you're even there for.**

Ready yourself with love and forgiveness. You have no idea what might be burdening another person. What fear, pain, or concern is hiding behind their insensitive words or behavior. Love your patients. Forgive them and forgive yourself. Eliminate judgment.

Patients or Customers?

Vince, a friend of mine, is an interesting individual. He's a pleasure to know and really fun to be around. He has an MBA and is smart, business savvy, charismatic, confident, a superb surgeon, and as a practicing urogynecologist, he exudes patient-centric excellence and professionalism. Yes, you are right, he's also handsome.

Vince runs a state-of-the-art pelvic floor and continence center, and he lives and dies by patient satisfaction and what he refers to as "the customer experience." The front desk, all providers and nurses, and his facility infrastructure and processes are all geared toward maximizing the customer experience and pleasing patients. Anything less—person, process, or issue—answers directly to Vince.

Initially, when Vince presented to me his philosophy of how he runs his practice, I thought he was nuts and pretty much told him so. Although we both share many common goals, including patient-centric excellence, I found his "customer service and satisfaction" speak annoying, and the opposite of what I write about and preach. Since then, I've given Vince's way further thought and consideration.

The patient-physician relationship is sacred and intimate, and it's based on a loving attitude, respect, trust, and forgiveness. It's what separates medicine from business. Corporate America has built an industry around commoditizing the patient-physician relationship. But the relationship is not a widget to be manufactured. I believe this devaluation and disrespect of our profession and relationship with patients is at the core of physician burnout.

Like Vince, my job is to provide patients with excellence, but it's not to make them satisfied or happy. My job is to respect them, to sacrifice for them, and to do everything possible to support their physical and emotional health. And as is the case with any personal relationship, healthy boundaries and expectations are important for both parties to thrive.

I didn't go to university for fourteen years and give my life to medicine to ensure that the mood music in the exam room is satisfactory or that the wait time is under a certain threshold. The next thing I'll be asked to provide is a greeter offering an iced latte, or perhaps a massage. I know of a hospital practice who actually cut down enormous trees in front of their building to accommodate patients who complained about the shaded waiting room. Unbelievable.

Remember, consultants peddle the belief that millions can be made advertising and boasting met metrics, hospital and provider rankings, and patient experiences. All under the guise of some noble mission of providing excellent care—to all of which I say, "Bull crap!"

If the patient is the customer, who in the hell am I? Their retail clerk, their waiter, their car wash attendant? I'm serious, who in the hell am I, and what do I get out of the deal? Especially when the relationship appears to be so one-sided. Do I get to fill out a physician satisfaction score regarding patient behavior? Do I get to complain or refuse to serve the customer when I'm not happy? What about *my* experience?

And finally, do the same consultants believe that teachers and parents should educate and raise the next generation with an even higher level of entitlement? To believe that the world exists solely to make them happy and satisfied? I have no doubt that if it makes money, the answer would be yes. And millions of others would follow suit, with no one thinking or certainly not admitting that it's all about the money.

In contrast to me, Vince actually believes that the customer experience is the holy grail, and his philosophy is not solely based on economics. His wiring truly believes that giving his patients a wonderful experience is an extension of his responsibility and calling to serve them as their physician. It's part of his DNA. His heartfelt love and respect for his patients, this environment he sets up is just a calling card on how it's delivered.

When I inquired after his thoughts regarding his philosophy and how it might pertain to burnout, I wasn't surprised by his answer. He truly believes it brings him joy, pride, and fulfillment when he prioritizes and optimizes the patient experience. Perhaps that's an interesting footnote to consider for those battling burnout.

So, patients or customers? Love, respect, trust, and forgiveness, or a commoditized transaction? A sacred intimate relationship, or a customer experience? Joy and fulfillment, or mood music and an iced latte? Or perhaps be like Vince; I think he has both.

TEAM TALK

Rude, entitled, and demanding patients stress all providers. Being disrespected by them is affecting the joy in nurses and APPs. For those who are frustrated, discouraged, or resentful toward their patients, the four Rs can be helpful.

If you find yourself regularly in survival mode, it may be time to reflect and to change your mindset and behavior. Fueled by empathy, love, and forgiveness, you can proactively use your gifts and talents to help others and serve. Your soul loves it when it has been nourished.

A JOURNEY MOMENT

Do you sometimes go into survival mode or distance yourself from patients when interacting with them? If yes, at day's end, are your emotions positive or negative?

_____

_____

_____

_____

_____

Do you think adopting the four Rs into your relationship with patients would be beneficial? If yes, write down a few ways of doing so.

1. _____
   _____
   _____

2. _____
   _____
   _____

3. _____
   _____
   _____

And lastly, do you serve patients or customers?

_____
_____
_____
_____
_____
_____

Chapter 25

Canadianizing the American Healthcare System? Forget About It!

As a Canadian who has lived and worked in a number of countries, I'm often asked about socialized healthcare. Recognizing the greed virus and how it's negatively impacted our healthcare system, I can appreciate why many are looking for other solutions. Recently, it's commonplace to hear someone arguing for a public-based system or Medicare for all. My thoughts regarding the matter have been consistent. My opinion has never wavered . . .

Forget about it. It's not going to happen. **Canadianizing the American healthcare system is never going to happen. The chance of this happening approaches impossible.**

America is a country controlled by money, power, and capitalism. In this country, patients want the best care and they want it now. We've been spoiled by tremendous access to a commodity named healthcare, and we don't mind blaming others when things go a little bit sideways. With a national debt of over $30 trillion, we have little flexibility regarding healthcare.

Good, bad, or indifferent, whatever you think about the American doctrine, our way of life is going to continue and not yield to a socialized system. Medical socialism is the antithesis of our American philosophy.

Scott MacDiarmid, MD

Let Me Explain

There's no question that from a philosophical standpoint it's a riveting debate whether or not the U.S. would be better served with a public healthcare system versus the private one we currently enjoy. Although I personally could endorse a government-based system, I don't think the average American advocating for one really understands how the system truly functions and its consequences. Let me explain.

All citizens and permanent residents of Canada receive Medicare, which is a publicly funded, single-payer universal healthcare system. Canadian hospitals are government-owned, similar to our Veterans Administration, meaning they don't make money, they only spend it. Canadians can purchase supplemental private insurance for services that aren't covered by Medicare, including dental, private rooms, and some medications. Otherwise, with few exceptions, there's no additional private option.

Medical litigation does exist, but it's a mere fraction of ours, and it's not part of the culture. For the majority of Canadians, suing your doctor is totally off their radar; taking personal responsibility and forgiveness rule the day. There is more of a cultural acceptance of good intentions and less judgment on outcome. As mentioned before, medications are less expensive as a result of government negotiations with U.S. manufacturers, otherwise certain medications may be excluded from formularies.

Everyone has free access to healthcare. It's paid for by taxes. Medications are cheaper. Litigation attorneys are looked down upon. Nobody goes bankrupt because of medical debt. And Canucks say, eh! Perfect, that sounds great, let's do it. But wait a minute, there's more.

Metaphorically, the elephant in the room is the obvious problem or difficult situation that people don't want to admit or talk about. When it comes to socializing the American healthcare system, there are a number of elephants; these elephants can't fly and never will.

Politicians and pundits who paint only one side of the story and pretend

244

that the elephants of a socialized healthcare system don't exist are ill-informed, naïve, or once again are just being deceitful.

So, let's get started. Let's speak to the four most obvious elephants in the room as it pertains to socializing medicine in the greatest country in the world who spends the most on healthcare.

We Won't Accept It

First and foremost, Americans will never accept long waits to see physicians and limited access to diagnostic tests and surgical procedures. In fact, it would throw our entitled culture into a ferocious tailspin.

A public-based healthcare system or socialized one is budget-based, not profit-driven. It lives and survives on revenues generated by taxes. It has an annual budget, much like your family. In order to meet the budget, access to care is limited, hospitals and hospital infrastructure are lacking, and there are not enough physicians to serve the public.

In Canada, it's normal to wait months, and I mean *months*, to see a primary care physician, and many of them no longer accept new patients. Recently, I referred my ex-mother-in-law to a fellow urologist in Montreal, but she couldn't get an appointment there for a year, so instead she flew to the Mayo Clinic in Rochester, Minnesota, and paid for the trip out of pocket.

It's the norm to wait months for a CT scan or an MRI, as the number of scanners are limited because of the budget. Most of the hospitals are aging, similar to U.S. public schools, with taxes unable to afford desperately needed new ones. And with limited private rooms available, how would you like to check into your local hospital and share a room with one to three other people?

Hospitals in Canada close entire floors during summer months and approaching year's end to save money and to meet the budget. Diagnostic tests and procedures routinely performed in offices in America are not permitted north of the border. They're performed only in hospitals and hospital clinics, where the government can bottleneck access and control cost. The lines are long when the burgers are cheap.

My sister's husband Andrew, a superb orthopedic surgeon in eastern Canada, has a two-year waiting list for elective surgery. That's a long time to wait when you're in pain needing a joint replacement. And that's on top of the six to twelve months just to see him for your initial consultation. When he orders an X-ray, once again you have to get in line.

Andrew takes two months off every summer when the hospital cuts his operating time to four hours a week, basically bringing his surgical practice to a temporary standstill. He has considered hiring recent orthopedic graduates as locum tenens who otherwise are unemployed, because the government is limiting billing numbers to new surgeons because they can't afford more. I repeat: newly trained physicians have no jobs because the government doesn't have the money to hire them.

When I finished my reconstructive fellowship at Duke in 1994, there was only one other surgeon with my expertise in Canada. In spite of this, I could not be offered an academic job in any university hospital because billing numbers were restricted. Hence, I stayed south, and here I remain today.

No, there aren't so-called death panels in Canada, but access to expensive specialized procedures and surgery is limited. For instance, my dad had to be medically evaluated before undergoing life-saving heart surgery. His surgeon explained to me that they are only budgeted for so many specialized cardiac procedures, and he could only offer the surgery to the healthier patients who had better odds of surviving. Although Dad passed the grade, he unfortunately died during the several weeks he was waiting for the procedure. (I love you, Dad, I miss you.)

My best friend, "no class" Johnny Grass I call him, injured his heart after being launched from his snowmobile that can travel at 115 miles an hour. Built like a Greek god, his enormous chest took the initial blow, likely saving his life, whereas a mere mortal like myself may have disintegrated. Johnny eventually needed a cardiac ablation to normalize his resultant highly symptomatic arrhythmia. After failing a number of cardioversions, he was placed on a twenty-two-month waitlist and strongly considered having it performed in South Carolina out of pocket.

Are you getting the picture? These personal stories are not cherry-picked, they are reality. It's what I grew up with. It's what I and other Canadians accept and quite frankly, do just fine with. And it may support why I believe Canadians are less entitled and more tolerant of their fellow man than the average American.

Look, the reason we have turbo-charged access to healthcare in the U.S. is because capitalism prints money providing it. We have endless scanners, because scanners make money. Your hospital is expanding at warp speed because bigger is profitable. You and your health are now a commodity, because your healthcare makes others rich. But remember, someone has to pay for it, and there's no free lunch.

I believe that socialized healthcare would throw our entitled "I want it now" culture into a ferocious tailspin. The limited access associated with a budget-based healthcare system will never happen in America; it's absolutely impossible. The elephant in the room is limited access, and it will never fly; we won't accept it.

We Can't Afford It

Unfortunately, the U.S. could never afford a public-based healthcare system and continue to provide its current level of access. The tax base could never support it. While it might have been attainable a few decades ago, our national debt now is much too high.

What you need to understand is that our same turbo-charged system, if delivered in Canada, would eventually bankrupt the nation. It's the reason why their care is limited. Whether you like it or not, you can't have your cake and eat it too.

And only the naïve or ill-informed argue that the system would be affordable by raising taxes or ending an unnecessary war. Of course that might help temporarily, but it won't be enough. Eventually we'll outgrow the new budget, and as always, our government will waste much of the money on other endeavors.

The bottom line is that we cannot afford our current commoditized access if it was paid for solely by taxes. The elephant in the room that we can't afford it is a sad reality.

It Will Tank the Economy

If somehow taxes could support a highly accessible and affordable healthcare system, what would happen to third-party payers, the makers of drugs and equipment, and your local hospital and physicians? What would happen to one-sixth of the economy?

Medicare and Medicaid don't reimburse enough for hospitals and private physicians to be viable. Their financial health is highly dependent on the fact that private insurance reimbursements keep hospitals and doctors solvent. Many hospitals actually lose money on Medicare patients, and many private physicians could never survive on that pay. The new oncology center, replacing the aging MRI scanner, expanding the emergency department—how would this happen if they were no longer significant profit centers? As the largest employer in many cities, a hospital system no longer making money would have an enormous negative impact on the financial health of the community.

Lowering the price of drugs and equipment associated with a public system would have enormous consequences. Less profitable and downsized pharmaceutical companies will hire fewer people and of course pay them less. They will spend less on bricks and mortar corporate infrastructure adversely affecting the economy. And the impact on the economy by gutting the insurance industry will be dramatic—remember that BlueCross and others spend a lot of money and employ a lot of people.

Medicare and Medicaid can't support the profit centers of the American healthcare system. It's the elephant in the room and financially hurting the Wall Street of medicine that will tank the economy.

Capitalism Wins

Whether you agree with me or not on my previous points, there's a fourth elephant in the room that I believe cements my position: capitalism wins. It doesn't matter what you and I may think, capitalism and the ruling class control this country, and they will never allow a socialized healthcare system.

The U.S. is run by money, by power, and it is controlled by the ruling class, regardless of party affiliation. Remember, money and lobbyists win, and we lose. The capitalists and government are not rolling over and giving up money, power, and control for the betterment of the country. The last time I looked, they're doing just fine.

A Few Predictions

When it comes to a country's healthcare system, there's no perfect solution. There's no magic formula or crystal ball to predict the future. But I think the future of our healthcare system and the financial health of our nation doesn't look good. Allow me to make a few predictions of what I see happening in the next decade.

I think that our healthcare system, for the most part, will continue to limp along in its current state. The Wall Street of medicine will print money, the government will bow down to lobbyists, and politicians will tell their constituents that they actually care.

I predict within two to three election cycles, politicians will start promising subsidies to help individuals afford their ever-increasing private payer premiums and deductibles. Let's face it, the rates are insane and compounding increases are devastating to many. It will become front and center as a voting issue.

The government will subsidize the system. It will selectively help individuals and industries who are either most in need, or the ones that will provide the most votes in doing so. As it did with higher education, government assistance will drive up costs further, and those supplying the commodity will profit even more. Remember the rule: keep the voter happy; votes and winning are what's important.

I think that Medicare and Medicaid will expand; they have to as our population ages and gets poorer relative to the cost of living. The expansion will be modest at best, but enough to support bragging rights to the voting public. The national debt will continue to rise, politicians will finger-point and blame, but our debt will increase, regardless of who's in power.

Sadly, there will always be the uninsured and those without coverage. This is a sad testimony to the greatest country in the world who spends the most on healthcare. The government is well aware that they can't afford to provide Medicare and Medicaid to the currently uninsured, otherwise they would have done so years ago.

I can envision that if government-sponsored healthcare does expand significantly, it will utilize the insurance industry, hospitals, and the private sector to do so. Remember, the government isn't good at running anything.

Basically, they'll hire the Wall Street of medicine, offering them highly lucrative programs supplying healthcare to millions, but under the guise of a government-based system. The same people will win, there will be plenty of losers, and debt will escalate.

But remember, a system that encourages patients to drop private insurance for a more affordable government option is not good for third-party payers, hospitals, and the makers of drugs and equipment. And the power of Wall Street is not going to allow this to happen.

Too Much Access and Too Much Profit

The bottom line is that there are two fundamental problems with the American healthcare system: *there is too much access and too much profit. Period.*

The system and government will never admit it. In fact, most everyone is recommending and encouraging higher access, and this will drive up cost and profit even further. And the average consumer, who is now spoiled and entitled, will further up their demands, throwing fuel on the fire.

The bottom line is that the Wall Street of medicine is making too much money and we can't afford it; access to healthcare needs to slow down because we are going broke; and the patient needs to rethink and lower their expectations, because they are not attainable.

Which leaves me with the biggest elephant in the room of all. The elephant of too much access and too much profit. We can't afford this elephant and it's not sustainable. This elephant just can't fly. But unfortunately people will never want less access, and business will never want less profit. So solutions to our current impasse are, for the moment, completely beyond me. I hope one day we can figure out a way for more people to access quality care for less money.

Team Talk

It's my belief that nurse burnout is less common in Canada versus the U.S. Nurses are not commoditized there and the profession is still respected. The goal of hospitals is to deliver healthcare with no emphasis being placed on making money.

The number of advanced practice providers is miniscule in Canada, but more are being trained, especially in the last decade. The government has been reluctant to graduate more primary care providers in its attempts to control cost. Increased access to healthcare would benefit most Canadians, but it's more expensive to deliver.

Ironically, immigrating to Canada as a U.S.-trained nurse or APP is actually a viable option for some. Whether or not practicing north of the border is more joyful and fulfilling is too complex to predict. Having said that, as long as you like cold weather, snowballs, and beer, I think that you would love living and practicing there, eh!

A Journey Moment

The pursuit of higher access and profit is promoting physician burnout. More, more, more. There's no end to the "more" madness. "More" is driven by corporatized healthcare and by many physicians' own choices and behavior. The elephant in the room is trumpeting, but very few are listening.

If you are suffering from burnout, is "more" adding to your problem? If yes, provide up to five ways it is doing so.

1. _____
2. _____
3. _____
4. _____
5. _____

Part 4: Finishing Strong

CHAPTER 26

THE MIND AND HEART OF A WARRIOR

My journey to find joy as a practicing physician has been a challenging but rewarding adventure. The climb to the summit has certainly had its ups and downs. One day I feel energized, proudly serving others, and the next day I am overwhelmed, fatigued, and sometimes even discouraged. I fluctuate between enjoying my interactions with patients to being angered and frustrated by their endless demands and unrealistic expectations. Today, I'm all in and could practice forever. Tomorrow, I yearn to be retired and think of possible exit strategies. So many different thoughts. So many different emotions.

It's interesting how quickly your thoughts can change, which then affects your emotions. Your emotions then fuel your words and actions. **Where your mind and thoughts go, your destiny will eventually follow.** Importantly, how you think impacts your ability to climb and to successfully reach your mountaintop.

In my struggle, I realized that the primary battle against burnout was not with my circumstances, with my patients, or with commoditized healthcare, which are generally ongoing and unchanging. But that the true battlefield where the most important battles are won or lost is in my mind. The battle is in my thoughts and how I choose to think from moment to moment.

For years I've been plagued by too much negative thinking regarding my job. I dwelled too much, ruminating over and over the multiple problems with healthcare. My toxic thinking became a source of my negativity, manifested by sarcastic or criticizing words and sometimes actions, which all pulled me back toward the valley of burnout and stole my joy.

You may not be able to control your circumstances, but you can control how you think about them. I got sick and tired of allowing my circumstances to make me feel unhappy, so I decided to make a life-altering change. I decided to change the way I was thinking and to develop what I call "the mind of a warrior." Having a mind of a warrior equips you to prevent or to battle burnout, and makes you a better climber within all life's domains. A well-prepared mind minimizes your slips and falls, and makes you more resilient to the difficulties experienced during your ascent to the summit. Training your mind is not easy. It takes time and discipline, but the rewards are great.

I was purposeful. I was proactive. I studied and developed new skills that have been very beneficial.

Let me share with you four ways to change your thinking and to develop the mind of a warrior.

Cognitive Reframing

We have already spoken briefly regarding cognitive reframing. It's a popular psychological technique used to shift your mindset so you're able to view a situation or person from a slightly different perspective. Creating a different way of looking at something changes its meaning, which can then affect thinking and behavior. You may not be able to control what happens, but you can control how you frame it.

By altering perception, reframing relieves stress and creates more positivity, independent of circumstances. It can change the physical and emotional responses to stress that are triggered by perceived stress, as well as by actual events.

When you catch yourself slipping into negative and stress-inducing thinking, ask yourself: What are some other ways to interpret the same information? Instead of seeing things the way you always have, challenge every negative thought, and see if you can adopt thoughts that fit your situation but reflect a more positive outlook.

The following steps will help you reframe.

Be Aware

The first step in reframing is to be aware of your negative thinking and any destructive thought patterns that may be burdening you. Self-awareness opens the door to addressing the problem.

Many physicians who are overwhelmed and stressed "learn" to become negative. Their chronic negative circumstances induce negative thinking that over time becomes ingrained, habitual, and more easily triggered. As the process self-propagates, we begin filtering work through a pessimistic lens, glossing over positive events while holding a magnifying glass to the negative. We start underappreciating what is functioning well and dwell on the stumbles and miscues. I am guilty as charged.

Having destructive thought patterns compounds the problem. Many of us overgeneralize and take isolated events and assume that all future events will be the same. Others become all-or-nothing thinkers, using words like *always* and *never* when describing things. For example, overgeneralizing that all patients are demanding, or thinking that patients can never be satisfied, are not beneficial thought patterns.

Know Your Triggers

I have a number of triggers at work that can easily set off my negative thinking. Once my stress response is triggered, I can become annoyed and angry, dwelling on the issue for hours afterward.

It's important to examine these triggers and your response when you are calm and not stressed. Ask yourself: Are my thoughts even true? And are there more positive ways to look at the situation that are less harmful to me?

For instance, I used to have a low tolerance for inadequate nursing care, especially in the hospital. Poor patient care could spark a cascade of negative thinking in me, as well as emotions, and sometimes I'd complain to others.

With introspection, the truth is that the majority of nurses do an excellent job; they work under challenging circumstances. Poor nursing care is the exception and not the rule. I now reframe these events as an opportunity to demonstrate patience or to constructively educate the nursing staff. This one simple reframe has helped me build character and in some cases benefits others.

Notice

Notice when your mind starts to wander into the sphere of negative thinking. Notice when your voice becomes firm or changes tone, your smile is gone, and your eyebrows are no longer happily spaced apart. The earlier that you recognize your emotional and physical responses to stress the better. It is easier to nip your negativity in the bud before it gains momentum and your blood begins to boil.

Pivot to Positivity

When you notice negative thinking, immediately pivot to positive thoughts and words. Substitute your thoughts with more positive ones, and change your self-talk to use less strong and negative emotions.

When looking at a potentially stressful situation, see if you can reframe it as a challenge versus a threat. Look for the gift in each stressful circumstance, viewing it in a way that still fits the facts of the situation, but is less negative and more optimistic and positive. And when needed, take a time-out and walk away for a few moments. Resist the soapbox; it brings everyone down.

Reward

Effective reframing will equip you as you develop a mind of a warrior. With a warrior's mind you will be more able to forgive, demonstrate self-control, and see the world's beauty and positivity, in spite of its imperfections.

Each time you reframe and feel its positive impact, give yourself a congratulatory fist pump. Self-reward encourages and energizes. At base camp, reevaluate your reframing successes and failures. It's a long journey to the summit and mastering this technique will make you a better climber.

Enrich Your Mind

The way we think is far more powerful than we often realize, and it impacts every aspect of our existence—either positively or negatively. Our relationships; finances; our emotional, physical, and spiritual health; how we function at work and find joy there; and our ability to enjoy life are all impacted by our thoughts.

Too often, I meditate on whatever spontaneously enters my mind, and in many cases my thinking is negative and nonproductive. I dwell on problems, making them appear to be larger and more difficult than they really are. I have a bad habit of overanalyzing and thinking about what can go wrong and envisioning the worst-case scenario. All these negative thoughts produce negative emotions, words, and actions. Remember, where your thoughts go your life follows.

The good news is that we have the choice on how to think, no matter what circumstances or situations we find ourselves in. Choose to enrich your mind to think positively toward every situation. The more positive you are the more powerful you will be.

Enriching your mind is a three-step process.

Say No to the Negative

Growing up I remember my mom regularly saying, "No, I'm not going to think about that." Having survived cancer, she was determined and disciplined not to be negative, fearing that negativity could jeopardize her emotional and physical health. Still enjoying her life thirty years later, it continues to be a successful strategy. (Love you, Mom!)

In order to have a mind of a warrior, it's important to say no to negative thinking. As soon as your thoughts wander into negative territory, say no and cast them aside. Stating that out loud is beneficial. Refusing to think about your endless problems will significantly reduce your negative emotions.

Replace with the Positive

To enrich your mind, it's important to replace negative thoughts with positive ones. Replace fear, worry, anger, and frustration with thoughts that are encouraging, loving, gentle, and grateful. Think about helping others and not focusing on your own problems.

Effective replacement will elevate you and those around you. Your positive warrior's mind will defend you from being pulled down by the much too pervasive consciousness of negativity.

Overwhelm with Good

Overwhelming and filling your mind with good and positive thoughts is one of the best ways to prevent negative thinking. Don't be a quiet bystander or take things for granted. Proactively think about the good and positive aspects of your life, including your family, friends, community, work, and your mental, spiritual, and physical health. Overwhelming and filling your mind with love, beauty, laughter, and what is good will allow little space for negativity.

It's important to be intentional and disciplined. Write down your positive thoughts and regularly voice them. Placing them in view will provide you with positive daily reminders.

Pre-Framing

Pre-framing is a technique that allows you to shape your thoughts about an event or situation prior to it occurring. It enables you to choose how to view or frame something before it even happens. It's especially helpful in reducing stress when the stressors are frequent, come on suddenly, and are relatively predictable.

At the end of this chapter, we will practice using pre-framing for some common stressful triggers we encounter as practicing physicians. Like a well-trained athlete, careful preparation on how we choose to pre-frame each trigger will reduce stress and better prepare us for the battle.

Make Declarations

Making a declaration creates a commitment. The commitment not only produces a new possibility for yourself, it generates something that you now have to move toward.

Declarations direct our lives toward what we speak. Like a small rudder guiding a ship in the direction that the pilot desires, our voice is a powerful tool that can help direct our path to the summit. The more specific the declarations are, the more powerful and effective they will be.

Be creative in making declarations that are both directive and inspiring. Base them on truth and don't minimize the power of any positive emotions that they may evoke. Be courageous, since the journey it may take you on could be life-changing.

Write down your declarations, memorize them, and recite them over and over. Repetition will prepare your mind and make you a better warrior.

Find Your Source

It's difficult to reframe, enrich your mind, pre-frame, and make affirming declarations day after day in the midst of the battle. It's challenging to have a positive warrior's mindset when the negatives associated with practicing medicine come so frequently and intensely.

I believe that in order to have a warrior's mind, you first need a warrior's heart. The heart of a warrior is a heart of love, gratefulness, forgiveness, humility, patience, and self-control.

Many need a source to provide them with the strength and fortitude to have a heart of a warrior. Some rely on their internal strength to pull them up toward their mountaintop, while others like me need a transcendent source. I rely on the grace of God, whose outstretched arm is always present, waiting to pull me upward.

I became a believer decades ago during a low point in my life, and as a result of my wife's unconditional love for me. Andrea made me realize that handing over the control of my life to Jesus Christ and relinquishing self-control was life-giving. "Let go let God" made so much sense, and at the time, it seemed so easy.

But over the years, I continued to live too much of my life relying on my own power and not the Lord's. Even though I love Christ and have a personal relationship with Him, I stubbornly tried to live my life my way and not His. As a consequence, I lived too many days fighting burnout and feeling discouraged, frustrated, tired, and angry.

Having a source will help you live life with a heart of a warrior. I know that the Holy Spirit and God's grace can provide me with infinite power to live joyfully and to reach my summit. The battles will continue, but great victories will be achieved.

Find your source, my friend—the summit is worth it.

Let's Practice Pre-Framing with a Mind and Heart of a Warrior

Let's evaluate a number of common stressors at work. We will examine their truth and proactively pre-frame each one with a more loving and forgiving spirit. We will write down affirming declarations and rehearse them over and over. And finally, by doing so we will live our thoughts and enjoy the beauty and grace experienced while living on the summit.

The Difficult Patient

Some of our patients appear ungrateful, demanding, rude, or even angry. Others are pressured and anxious, or have unrealistic expectations that make treating them difficult. They generate a lot of stress and unhappiness for physicians and staff. With a stroke of a pen they can demoralize us by giving us a low patient satisfaction score or with cruel words written on social media. Their attitude and actions can threaten the sanctity of the patient-physician relationship and foster physician burnout.

When we evaluate difficult patients, a number of truths can be established. Most of our patients are kind, respectful, thankful, and value us, even if they don't outwardly show it. Difficult patients represent a small percentage of cases, but their effect on us can be great.

When we encounter difficult people, we don't know what they may be going through, acutely or ongoing. Many are under a lot of physical, emotional, or financial stress, and we might be interacting with them during a bad day where they have encountered wait times, traffic, parking, staff, and our own behavior may also have given them a legitimate reason to be upset.

Stressed and difficult patients are here to stay, but fortunately we get to choose how we interact with them. Getting upset and going home frustrated and angry is not a good strategy and only makes your emotional state worse. Letting unfavorable reviews irritate you and make you bitter is an enormous self-inflicted wound.

It's entirely possible that we have all been "the difficult patient" to someone else, perhaps not as a patient, but when interacting with others. How many times have you barked at a waiter or customer assistance when you are stressed or angry? And all of us wish that we could be forgiven and treated kindly, even when we are least deserving.

With the heart of a warrior, we can reframe the difficult patient. We can see them through a lens of love, empathy, and forgiveness, enabling us to make bold declarations as their provider. Make the following declarations and recite them over and over. Write it, say it, and live it daily.

"I choose to treat each and every patient with a loving and forgiving spirit."

"I will care for my patients as I would want them to care for me."

"I have the strength, the discipline, and willpower to serve my patients nobly, regardless of how I am treated or how I feel."

"When I slip and fall, I will lift myself up and continue to serve. I will not fail—my purpose is too important."

Relying on a transcendent source, my personal declarations are:

"I will honor God by choosing to treat each and every patient with a loving and forgiving spirit."

"I will love and care for my patients as God loves and cares for me."

"The Holy Spirit provides me the strength, the discipline, and will power to serve my patients nobly, regardless of how I am treated or how I feel."

"When I slip and fall, God will lift me up and carry me on my journey to serve. I will not fail—with God I have already won."

Inadequate Staff

Too often physicians are like restaurant owners trying to provide a wonderful dining experience to customers with not enough capable staff. We are trying to deliver excellent care with a fragmented team that in many cases is not capable or interested in the mission. When the buck stops with us, it's difficult to work in this environment. Herding cats is a regular source of frustration, anger, and physician burnout.

The truth is that it's easy to criticize the quality of healthcare delivery, but it is a complicated matter that is difficult to address. The causes are multifactorial and, in many cases, the underlying problems are worsening. Many staff and nurses are overworked, underpaid, and underappreciated by patients, physicians, and by healthcare systems. They are stressed from hitting endless roadblocks—unpredictable patient scheduling, frustrating insurance calls, and constant demands by patients and supervisors. Others are inexperienced, undertrained, not kept accountable, and on-the-job training and encouragement is lacking. It's difficult to be excellent in the trenches of commoditized healthcare, when arguably there is not much in it for them.

I know that my expectations are too high and unrealistic when it comes to the performance of others. Judging others based on personal standards often results in frustration, criticism, and negativity. Working with a fragmented team is difficult, but the good news is that we get to choose how we think and respond to this stressful reality.

With a warrior's heart, we can reframe workforce challenges through the lens of understanding, patience, and respect. Compassionately we can take responsibility to lead, lift up, and empower others. As a warrior, repeat the following declarations over and over and victory will ensue:

"I choose to treat my staff and nurses with compassion and respect."

"In the heat of the moment, I will be patient and understanding."

"I will empower and encourage my staff and nurses to use their gifts and talents to serve and to enjoy the fruits of their difficult labor."

"It is my responsibility to lead and train the healthcare team, to hold them accountable, and to make them feel appreciated and proud."

"My success will be measured by my effort and by bettering others."

My personal declarations:

"I choose to honor God and to treat my staff and nurses with compassion and respect."

"In the heat of the moment, the Holy Spirit will provide me the strength to be patient and understanding."

"The Holy Spirit will help me empower and encourage others to use their gifts and talents to serve and to enjoy the fruits of their difficult labor."

"It is my responsibility to honor God by leading and training the healthcare team, by holding them accountable, and by making them feel appreciated and proud."

"My success will be measured by my effort, by bettering others, and by pleasing God."

Death by a Thousand Cuts

Today's healthcare system is like a death by a thousand cuts. Electronic medical records have burdened us with endless clerical duties and tasks, adversely affecting patient care and promoting burnout. Government and third-party payers have beaten us down with rules, regulations, and pre-authorizations. Some days it seems impossible not to be annoyed, frustrated, and discouraged.

The truth is that our healthcare system is much too complex to even consider going back to paper charts. EMR should be more user-friendly, yet it provides countless efficiencies and has helped revolutionize patient care. For those who remember going to the medical record department to sign their hospital charts, thank goodness those days are over.

The healthcare system represents one-sixth of the economy, and it needs to be paid for and regulated. We could pontificate about the appropriate roles of third-party payers and government in healthcare, but they are both here to stay, and their perceived negatives are likely going to persist or worsen.

With a heart of a warrior we can choose to reframe death by a thousand cuts through the lens of understanding, acceptance, and perseverance, and to make powerful and affirming declarations. Proactively make the following declarations when you feel frustrated:

"I choose to accept the burdens of practicing medicine to help others."

"Feeling annoyed and frustrated reminds me of my privilege to serve."

"I will persevere through my feelings because my mission is too important."

My personal declarations:

"I choose to accept the burdens of practicing medicine to help others and to honor God."

"Feeling annoyed and frustrated reminds me of the privilege God gave me to serve."

"God gives me the strength to persevere through my feelings, because His mission for me is too important."

Overworked

There is wear and tear on the minds and bodies of physicians from habitually overworking. We get up early, come home late, and multitask throughout the day under stressful circumstances. The pressure, responsibility, and being on call can weaken even the strongest. Many physicians feel overwhelmed and exhausted, and the ill effects from overworking increases the propensity for burnout.

Being overworked is poorly defined and subjective. The truth is that caring for patients is mentally and physically challenging, but many of the wounds we experience from being overworked are self-inflicted.

Until recently, no one has made physicians work long hours and at such a pace. Although many now have employers dictating their schedule, our overwork culture has always been part of the profession. Patient care is demanding, but ego, greed, pride, habit, patient needs, and expectations are other factors driving our conscientiousness to work even harder. Just think how many physicians feel guilty when their day is not jammed full. Yes, physicians are an interesting breed.

With the heart of a warrior, we can reframe our work through the lens of love and wisdom and choose to live more joyfully. The love for our family, friends, community, and for our personal health can help us prioritize what's important and help us live a more balanced life. Wisdom will teach us to love and live more and to work less. Having a warrior's heart, and with love and wisdom, recite the following declarations over and over:

"Being tired reminds me that I was called to be a physician."

"I have the strength to endure and the wisdom to rest."

"Wisdom and love for my family says it's been a good day. It's time to go home—I have had enough."

"I choose my family, relationships, and health over work and money."

My personal declarations:

"Being tired reminds me that God called me to be a physician."

"God provides me the strength to endure and the wisdom to rest."

"Wisdom and love for my family says it's been a good day. Thank you, God. It's time to go home—I have had enough."

"I choose God, family, relationships, and health over work and money."

High-Pressure Medicine

Many procedures and operations physicians perform are high-pressure and stress-provoking. (This is not to diminish the stress associated with office-based medicine, but prescribing medication and counseling patients about lifestyle changes is generally less worrying.)

The truth is that surgery and procedures are not always successful, and they may result in significant complications. In our commoditized world of healthcare, patient expectations are increasingly high; many have little tolerance for imperfect outcomes or problems. The stress associated with these high expectations is causing burnout.

Over time, practicing such high-pressure medicine can instill fear into some providers. Just the thought of performing complicated surgery and its potential poor outcomes can elicit a visceral response. Even the most capable and confident can surrender to their thoughts and start avoiding risky procedures to lessen their exposure.

Fortunately, we get to choose our thoughts and how we frame these fearful stressors.

With a heart of a warrior, reframe your fear, anxiety, and worry through the lens of love, confidence, and faith. Your love for patients and your willingness to sacrifice for them will ease your worries. Have confidence that you have the gifts and talents to help patients; this will defeat your anxiety. Have faith that you are serving others, which will help eliminate your fear. Through the lens of love, confidence, and faith, repeat the following declarations:

"I will sacrifice for my patients and say no to fear."

"I was made to do what is difficult."

"Risk reminds me of my calling to serve others."
"I welcome worry and anxiousness if that is what it takes to help others."
"A difficult climb to the summit will make the views more spectacular."

My personal declarations:
"The Holy Spirit equips me to sacrifice for my patients and say no to fear."
"God made me to do what is difficult."
"Risk is God's reminder that He has called me to serve."
"I welcome worry and anxiousness if that is what it takes to serve God and to help others."
"A difficult climb to the summit will make God's beautiful views more spectacular."

Remember, where your thoughts go, your destiny and life will follow. Having a mind and heart of a warrior will equip you to control your thinking and make you a better climber. Finding your source will grant you love, gratefulness, forgiveness, humility, patience, and self-control. When you transform work from your battlefield to your mission field it will guarantee you success in reaching your summit.

Team Talk
Many nurses and APPs are plagued by too much negative thinking. Identify your stressors and commit yourself to the exercises outlined.

Remind yourself that hard work now will benefit you and others long term. Personalize your declarations, and don't be afraid to be courageous and emotional. Your declarations may be the gateway that will inspire and motivate.

Scott MacDiarmid, MD

A Journey Moment

Continue pre-framing by identifying other stressors that you commonly experience at work. Carefully examine their truth and pre-frame each through the lens of one having a heart of a warrior. Write down affirming declarations and recite them over and over. Think, write, say, and then live the new and exciting journey that you will take yourself on. When you have mastered work stressors, then move on to stressful triggers you encounter in other life domains including family, friends, community, and health.

I have given you a few other potential work stressors to help you get you started.

Partner Conflicts

_____

_____

_____

_____

_____

_____

_____

Administrator Woes

_____

_____

_____

_____

_____

_____

_____

Tight Finances

_____

_____

_____

_____

_____

_____

_____

Other Stressors

_____

_____

_____

_____

_____

_____

_____

Chapter 27

A Call to Action to Address Your Fear

Find a quiet spot, grab your favorite drink, sit back, and let's talk. If you've made it this far reading this book, we've likely formed somewhat of a trusting relationship. I want you to love practicing medicine and to live each day on your mountaintop. I desperately want you to feel joyful and fulfilled while serving and sacrificing for others. There's no higher calling, and the world needs you.

And with that goal in mind, this chapter is one of the most important. It's written to challenge you to think, to reflect, to write, and for some, to pray. It demands you to dig down deep into your soul and ask yourself some pretty tough questions. It challenges you to face your fears and make decisions for a successful future.

I want you to read this chapter when you have time to think! When you have time to reflect and write down some thoughts. Those written thoughts are a catalyst for an actionable game plan and strategy. Words that you can go back to later and rethink even further. Those words are the foundation for your journey. You will look back to them often, as you climb.

Don't underestimate the power of writing: it demands that you reflect, and it helps you begin to understand yourself. When words become a call to action, then personal joy and fulfillment will become a reality.

So, take a sip, and let's get started.

Addressing Your Fears

We have previously spoken about physician fear and how it relates to the greed virus. In order for many physicians to reach their mountaintop, they are going to have to address a number of fears by first answering some pretty tough questions. They are going to have to give up some things—some good, some bad—and take actionable steps to realize their true potential. Here are some questions to help you identify your fears.

Are you afraid of *losing income* if you were to give yourself that desperately needed margin by cutting back, by getting a scribe, or by doing one less case? Or will you continue to live fatigued and stressed, running even faster on the hamster wheel of corporatized healthcare?

Are you afraid of *losing control and perfection* by empowering others and keeping them accountable? Or will you continue to come in early and stay late, and answer the same task with the same answer, and hit "send" to the same person, day after day?

Are you afraid of *confrontation* with your partners or administrators, sharing with them the issue or issues that are just wearing you down? Will you continue to be silent, bitter, and resentful, going home at night to unload on your family?

Are you afraid of *saying no* to BlueCross, saying no to your hospital, and at times saying no to your patients? Or will you continue to live frustrated, discouraged, and even hopeless, like a puppet on a string?

Or are you afraid or perhaps too proud to *admit to yourself*, to your colleagues, to your family or employer, *that you're suffering*, that you're anxious, that you're burning out? And that maybe you need their help, their understanding, and perhaps their forgiveness? All might be necessary in order for you to climb out of your valley and begin the climb to your glorious mountaintop. That place of meaning and purpose. That place of finishing strong.

TEAM TALK

Nurses and APPs must also address various fears by answering questions and taking action in order to be joyful and fulfilled. I recommend for them to join physicians in doing the following Journey Moment and to modify it accordingly.

A JOURNEY MOMENT

Self-Analysis

Here's a simple self-analysis exercise that may be beneficial. Examine your fears and concerns, and grade each one's severity. Rank 0 (no concern) to 5 (paralyzing concern). Consider these and many others, and be honest with yourself; it's no time for denial and defense mechanisms.

Concern Scale

Fears	No				Paralyzing	
Losing income/security	0	1	2	3	4	5
Loss of control/perfection	0	1	2	3	4	5
Confrontation	0	1	2	3	4	5
Saying no	0	1	2	3	4	5
Admitting suffering	0	1	2	3	4	5
Other	0	1	2	3	4	5

Having completed this, jot down some ideas that address or describe each fear and concern. Remember that today's thoughts and writings are just the beginning of your new journey.

Then make courageous decisions to address each one. Write down thoughts that support and help turn your decisions into an actionable strategy. Start slowly, but step by step, make forward progress on your upward ascent to your mountaintop. Remember base camp.

Then in a few months, without looking at your original answers, repeat the same analysis. Monitor your progress. Fist pump your improvements. Continue to work on areas that need to be addressed. And remember, the greater the fear, the greater the stronghold on your joy and fulfillment, the greater the reward when positively impacted.

Fear and concern #1:

_____

_____

Decisions:

_____

_____

Actionable strategy:

_____

_____

Fear and concern #2:

_____

_____

Decisions:

_____

_____

Actionable strategy:

_____

_____

Fear and concern #3:

_____

_____

Decisions:

_____

_____

Actionable strategy:

_____

_____

Fear and concern #4:

_____

_____

Decisions:

_____

_____

Actionable strategy:

_____

_____

Fear and concern #5:

_____

_____

Decisions:

_____

_____

Actionable strategy:

_____

_____

My Personal Journey

I can honestly say that in the last few years I've made real progress addressing the five fears noted, as well as many others. Looking back, my journey began with the initial steps of realization, followed by the early climb of acceptance. Then finally and most importantly, I took a number of brave and difficult upward steps of positive and impactful decisions, always looking up, always climbing.

For instance, I'm now pretty much at peace with my financial security, and it's not based on net worth or potential future earnings. It's based on the decision that I'm no longer willing to sacrifice myself and my family's joy for money and security. I'm no longer willing to be burned out running faster on the hamster wheel for a few extra dollars. Although I still struggle with the temptation to make more money, it's liberating to abandon such fears, and the resulting peace is priceless.

I sometimes laugh regarding my conscious decision to no longer be such a perfectionist. I've always been proud of being one, since I believe it drives excellence. But giving up just a bit of this tendency, I've found it surprisingly freeing and less stressful. I laugh when I acknowledge that I'm letting something go, while in other situations I still hold the line. And remember, I've corporatized my clinic. I've deputized my nurse, Jenna. I've empowered others. Fist pumps.

I now stand up for myself so much better than I used to. An alpha male in my younger years, it's surprising how much I now avoid confrontation; in fact it's a weakness. Realizing this, I recently made a good decision to no longer be pushed around by colleagues or administrators in the workplace. I made a decision to speak up, and when needed, appropriately push back.

Those who push are often sneaky, self-righteous, or passive aggressive, the masters of projection; others are insecure bullies or just plain mean. Of course, I give grace and carefully pick my battles, but I'm ready to push back at a moment's notice. And it's funny how the "bullies" get quieter and less aggressive once they realize your willingness to defend your ground. The result? It's now rare for me to go home at day's end stewing and taking out frustrations on my family.

I decided and learned to set up healthy boundaries, especially with patients. I initially overshot the mission and had to tone down my survival mode tactics: abruptness and firmness. Although I'm a work in progress, I'm now pretty good at gently saying no to the patient tail wagging the physician dog. And my nurses have followed suit and are similarly benefitting. Balancing empathy with appropriate patient expectations and boundaries has really helped me enjoy my job and my patient-physician relationships.

And finally, realizing and admitting that I was burned out—filled with a heart of bitterness and resentment—was the most important step in my recovery. Again, when my wife and daughter lovingly called me out on it, and after getting off my knees in prayerful reflection, I then decided that I was on a new and exciting journey to my mountaintop that will go on forever. I decided to do anything necessary to achieve my goal and to better my life with them. *Nothing* is more important to me than Andrea and Lindsey.

It's been a life-giving journey of decisions; some of them have been pretty tough, but the ongoing climb to my summit is such a blessing.

CHAPTER 28

SEE THE SUMMIT BY SERVING

Most of us know the work of Stephen R. Covey, famous for authoring the book *The 7 Habits of Highly Effective People.* In 1996, *Time* magazine named him one of the twenty-five most influential people, and his words and wisdom truly stand the test of time.

I want to bring into our discussion his second habit, "Begin with the End in Mind." This habit is based on imagination, the ability to envision in your mind what your eyes cannot presently see. Covey believes that physical creation follows mental creation. And if you don't make a conscious effort to visualize who you are and what you want in life, then you allow others and circumstances to shape you and control your destiny.

As noted, I believe that those who envision their mountaintop, who define and see their summit, are far more likely to be successful in their journey. Those who see the summit and begin with the end in mind are great climbers. Envisioning the glorious view from the mountaintop empowers them, it encourages them, it's what gives them the discipline and strength to continue. It keeps them focused.

Experts instruct us to write down our goals and vision. In chapter 8, we defined our mountaintop for all five life domains: work, family, friends, community, and health (mental, spiritual, and physical). Go back and review them, and make any appropriate adjustments. Your goals should be clear and well-defined to yourself and to others. They should be measurable and have delivery dates. Target dates foster accountability as well as motivate. For example, "I'm going to lose weight" won't motivate you as much as "I'm going to lose fifteen pounds in six weeks."

Goals should also be realistic and attainable. For instance, deciding to leave work earlier to spend time with family by seeing four or five fewer patients daily or hiring a scribe in the next few months. Start a journey toward a new career by immediately beginning an online degree. Don't be afraid to take a chance, to learn a new skill, or to push yourself beyond comfort. Challenges can be life-giving and the growth in you will flourish even when you fall short of difficult objectives.

Make your written goals visible—on your desk, bathroom mirror, or computer—and review them often. Proactively address them with baby steps, each step taking you closer toward the summit. Great climbers know when to pivot, when to change direction. They anticipate changing landscapes and proactively make adjustments. The best are always looking up; they're always climbing with the end in mind.

But remember base camp. At day's end, or a few times a week, take stock. Ask yourself what you're doing well, what you're doing poorly, and what you need to work on. Evaluate your forward progress. Check your pace and check your direction. Unpack negative thinking, and remember, fist pump even the smallest of successes and accomplishments.

I'm a Dopamine Doer

"Listen freckle face, focus," I was told. The words came from an attorney preparing me for a medical legal case. I was fully engaged with her, but doing multiple other tasks simultaneously.

The lawyer wasn't the first to comment about my multitasking and restlessness. My mother-in-law once said, "The church sermon was wonderful, but Scott couldn't sit still." And for decades at meetings, my chair was always pushed back, always at table's end, and always closest to the exit and coffee.

Having attention deficit disorder, I struggle with the "begin with the end in mind" advice. Envisioning and writing down my summit, making a strategic plan—I'd never done this and just the thought of it makes me a little nervous, or vaguely overwhelmed; I'm not sure why.

I've always been a doer. In fact, a doer on steroids. I check tasks off my list daily, and that list is endless and keeps on growing. For the most part, my behavior explains much of my success because being conscientious and being highly productive are not the worst sins with which to be afflicted.

But I'm not a planner. I don't look far into my or my family's future. I think it's a significant weakness.

I think it explains why I've lived and found myself in certain places or circumstances that are less than ideal. I think it's why I'm currently struggling visualizing my exit strategy as I get older. When asked where do I want to live once retired and what that retirement might look like, my answer is pretty vague. Which is kind of sad for an otherwise disciplined and intentional soul.

The inability to begin with the end in mind for many may be partially related to brain wiring.

Those with attention deficit disorder struggle with planning. The ADD brain is under-stimulated and always hungry for reward. We're always looking for things we can do to get rewarded in the present moment, and the dopamine hit of satisfaction is endlessly addicting. We want to accomplish tasks in the present, because the future is always hazy, and may be irrelevant. And concentrating on mapping out a schedule or drawing up a detailed plan in advance, forget about it! Not appealing.

Dopamine is released in our brain when we achieve, not when we plan. As Andrea has told me: "The problem with living life as a dopamine doer is what happens when you're no longer capable of doing?" When you're no longer a physician. When you're no longer physically or mentally able to perform tasks that normally define you. Too many find themselves retired and asking, "Where am I and what can I do? Why am I here, and what am I worth? How do I find success? How do I find meaning?"

Yielding to Andrea's wisdom that planning is important, I was challenged to see my summit. And now that I'm more focused on the future, we can walk this journey together.

Am I Serving?

At first glance, Covey's words are readily applied to finite goals and materialism, but intentionally, they have a much deeper meaning and relate to one's identity and purpose.

Covey challenges us to envision our funerals, asking us what we want others to say about us, and give thought to who attends. Pause and think about this for a moment; it's a thought-provoking exercise.

I agree with Covey that to begin with the end in mind applies to every field of the human endeavor, including family, friends, work, community, and the different aspects of health. And also that we are the guardian and protector of our purpose and future. It's our ultimate responsibility.

I encourage each of you, when defining your mountaintop, to remember your purpose, to remember your why. In order to be fulfilled in your life's journey, it must extend far beyond finite goals and materialism.

It's essential to integrate your purpose "to serve" into all five life domains. Using your gifts and talents to serve others not only applies to patients. It applies to family, to friends, and to your community and yourself. We all have been blessed with so many gifts, and those gifts need to be shared with others. And every decision you make to serve, whether small or large, will shape and define your mountaintop of joy and fulfillment.

Serving family has generational impacts. Serving friends builds priceless memories and relationships. Serving community can be life-changing to so many. Serving and prioritizing your health will fuel and strengthen you. And serving your patients will nourish your soul as well as the world.

Every day, see the summit as an opportunity to serve. And no matter how small of a step, serving others in all domains will bring you one step further

along in your journey. One step closer to that glorious view from the summit. That glorious eternal view as a result of serving.

TEAM TALK

I encourage nurses and APPs to see the summit and to begin with the end in mind. I inspire them to remember their purpose and to serve others, not only at work but in all five life domains.

Be a mom or a dad and change the world by positively impacting the next generation.

Be a best friend or better still, comfort a stranger.

Get your mind off work and serve your community. Remember those wise words, "This is a job and not your life."

Go for a walk and exercise often. Sleep and rest. Put your physical, mental, and spiritual health at the front of the line. Fuel the engine that is needed to successfully climb to the summit.

Serving in all five life domains with the end in mind will nourish the soul that you have been blessed with. It will nourish the soul that was individually designed for you to impact others.

Please finish strong. The view from the summit is beautiful and everlasting.

A JOURNEY MOMENT

Once a week, or preferably more often, take a few moments and ask yourself: Am I serving? Think about all five life domains. Record the date or even better, use a calendar.

If yes, you're serving, jot down a few comments on how (and don't forget the fist pumps). If no, write down a strategy that might encourage you this week to do so. Use the calendar in this exercise for the next several weeks. Don't be surprised if you find yourself serving more as a result. Like gratitude and attitude, positive actions and emotions can be learned behaviors.

Serving Calendar:

Date:

See the Summit   Am I Serving?

Family	Yes	How:
	No	Strategy:
Friends	Yes	How:
	No	Strategy:
Community	Yes	How:
	No	Strategy:
Work	Yes	How:
	No	Strategy:
Health	Yes	How:
	No	Strategy:

CHAPTER 29

PEOPLE WHO SERVE: FACES OF FIRST RESPONDERS

I would like to finish our journey that we have taken together by honoring those who serve our community. I want to salute the men and women who work on the front lines—the nurses, the teachers, the military, the firefighters, the police, and others. I want to acknowledge and thank the first responders who get up each day to sacrifice and to help our nation. Serving others is rewarding but it's also difficult and burdensome. Unfortunately, too many of our first responders suffer from burnout.

The Front Lines

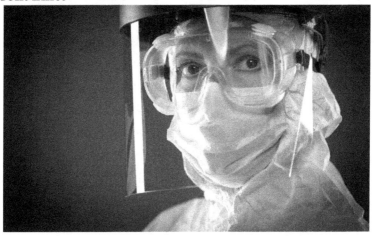

Photo credit: Feverpitched by iStock

In emergency departments nationwide, nurses battle on the front lines as highly skilled warriors caring for the seriously ill and dying patients.

It's on the front lines where nurses live and experience America. They see us at our best and have witnessed the worst—trust me. Chest paddles giving life to the lifeless. Bags of O negative blood rescuing a body broken from a head-on collision. Pulling a marble out of a child's throat, then gently handing her back to her grateful mom and dad. With excellence and dedication, the emergency room team are all in to lift up, to fix, and to cure the pain, fear, and illness in their community.

But the ER is not always life-giving. They can't always relieve the symptoms or stem the bleeding; they don't always get a thank-you. In fact, on the front line, nurses experience the opposite, daily.

Too often the aged heart is unable to beat another day; watching someone die is never easy. Obesity and diabetes are taking their toll, both diseases threatening the health of millions. Then there's the loss of civility—rudeness, patients yelling, even taking a swing at healthcare providers. Security gets called in. Tripped-out addicts, well-known to the staff, are readmitted, the needle marks their tattoo of hopelessness. On a bad night, the emergency department is not for the weak.

Early in her career, Jennifer was among the nurses who cared for the survivors of Hurricane Katrina that killed 1,833 people and left millions homeless in New Orleans. That's where she got her first taste of disaster relief, solidifying her love for emergency medicine. With love and a hunger to care for the acute and injured, Jennifer later volunteered as a front-line nurse in New York City for twelve weeks during the height of the pandemic in that city.

When I wrote this, the death toll that day in New York from the coronavirus was 779, the highest single-day total. The authorities were still optimistic that the curve was bending. When I thought of Jennifer and her safety, I hoped this was true.

She was driven by her calling to use her gifts and talents to help others, and Jennifer successfully battled the front lines with so many other healthcare providers. She safely returned home and rejoined her emergency room colleagues. I'm so proud of Jennifer for her bravery and willingness to serve. I am so proud of all nurses on the front lines and the millions of others throughout our healthcare system. To all, please be safe, and thank you for serving.

Another Cheer from Marilyn

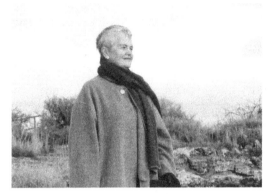

Family Photo

Marilyn is brilliant and gifted with giving. As a math wizard, Marilyn taught enriched math and calculus to high-school students for decades. She made calculations fun. She gave confidence to those with none. Her patience, her smile, her encouragement—day after day, all positive and infectious.

As a teacher pursuing her love and care for the underappreciated and less gifted, she introduced bridge to the public school system. She called it "mental gymnastics." To this day the curriculum flourishes, teaching a life-long skill and giving joy to so many.

Behind the scenes, Marilyn cared for and loved countless others. There was the boy with Tourette's syndrome to whom she gave the gift of friendship and pride. The young pregnant couple fighting poverty and addiction had their bills paid by her and she gave them gifts. She donated so many clothes, shoes, Christmas ornaments to the community, trading things she liked for the joy of giving.

Extroverted and opinionated, and often the vocal person in the room, Marilyn gave her time, her money, and her life gifting her soul to her students and to others. Serve, help, and smile. She says, "I care about you," "You can do it," "Believe in yourself."

My mom Marilyn is now ninety. She thinks often of her kids, her grandchildren, about social concerns, and more recently, politics. Smiling, contented, she's at peace for the most part.

With fingers and eyes fixated on her computer, she engages with others around the world playing bridge. As a grand master, she scores another win, another cheer to a deserving opponent, always another cheer from Marilyn.

She deserves the smile on her face, her contentment.

Mom, thank you for being one of the millions of teachers who love and sacrifice for their students and community. Generations are blessed by your profession.

A Thousand Words

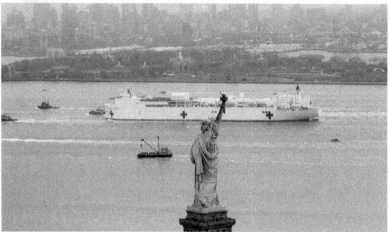

Photo credit: Mike Segar, Reuters

Standing strong she looked out to sea. Brave, stoic, on guard.

Behind her, the war raged. Millions affected, thousands dying, fear silencing the streets. Where is the help at a time like this? Where is the hope when bodies are mounting? You could see it in their eyes: *God please help us.*

The seas at her feet were thankfully calm. Wakes were modest and visible. Not surprisingly, the skies were gray but glimmers of brightness, of courage, of optimism and safety approached. There was even a light shining, perhaps a transcendent reminder that help was coming. Yes, in spite of the misery, there came an oasis of hands of care and comfort.

And then, there it stood. Greeted by her extended shining light cheering its presence. Massive white armor ready for battle. Armor protected by red shields of love and healing. Armor decorated by twelve hundred strong. Six feet apart they stood, the mist anointing their confidence, their discipline, their readiness to fight and to win. Yes, her light shone down on another mission to save a nation under siege.

A photo says a thousand words; this was taken on March 30, 2020 by Adam Jeffery, and I believe should be embedded in the mind and soul of every American.

To the U.S. military, I hold up my torch with its shining light. And as did Lady Liberty, I hold up my gratitude, my respect, and my freedom to every member of the military who serve our nation and to the USNS *Comfort*. Thank you and God bless you all.

The Heroes of 9/11

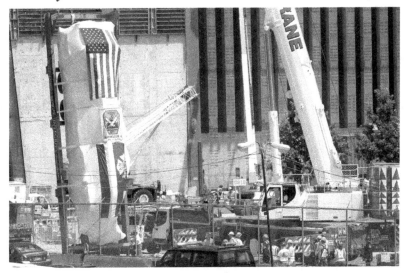

Photo credit: Mike Segar, Reuters

I was sitting in the chairman's office at the University of Alabama in Birmingham when the first plane hit. Knowing this, my interview for a faculty position immediately seemed awkward, almost irrelevant. Nearly three thousand people died on September 11, 2001, and the world changed forever.

With all planes grounded, I was sitting in the back of a town car taking me back to Memphis, wondering what in the heck just happened.

All of us have seen the footage. The Twin Towers of the World Trade Center collapsing into dust, the Pentagon wounded, and the field in Shanksville, Pennsylvania. We've seen the direct hits, we've seen the smoke and carnage, we've seen desperate souls jumping. The voices from the cockpit recorder of United Airlines Flight 93 I'll remember forever: "I don't want to die," "Are you ready?" and "Let's roll." It was a day that, around the world, we collectively bowed our heads as unbelievable heroism met unbelievable evil.

The attack on 9/11 is the single deadliest terrorist attack in human history, and 343 firefighters died as first responders. Ladder Company 3 took on some of the heaviest casualties, losing most of its men. Reporting to the North Tower, Captain Patrick "Paddy" Brown and his men were last known to be on the thirty-fifth floor.

Captain Paddy J. Brown, Lt. Kevin W. Donnelly, Michael Carroll, James Raymond Coyle, Gerard Dewan, Jeffrey John Giordano, Joseph Maloney, John Kevin McAvoy, Timothy Patrick McSweeney, Joseph J. Ogren, Steven John Olson, all victims of 9/11. All on board Ladder Company 3's fire truck fulfilling their duty to help and to save others.

Prior to 9/11, I never gave much thought to folks who served as firefighters. Growing up, I recall Jay's brother John being one. I remember others applying who were not accepted. Seemingly they were a good bunch of down-to-earth guys, handy, athletic, often they took second career jobs after an early retirement. But a "first responder" job as an inherently risky one? Those thoughts were not mine growing up in eastern Canada.

But my thoughts regarding firefighters and all first responders have changed forever. Ladder Company 3 fire truck has since been lowered into the National September 11 Memorial and Museum, a timeless reminder of their heroism and sacrifice. It's a timeless reminder of my appreciation.

The Thin Blue Line

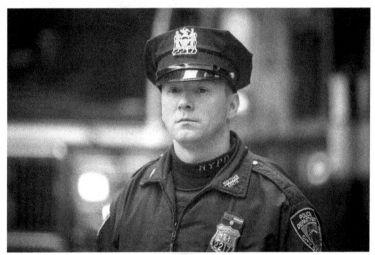

Photo credit: palinchakjr by iStock

Domestic violence. Heroin addicts selling on the street. A person beaten by six others because he was in the wrong place at the wrong time. A child kidnapped, agonized parents attending her funeral months later. A basement window just broken, and you're upstairs alone sleeping. We need help.

A drunk and angry driver swerving on the wrong side of the road with innocence ahead threatened. The local deli robbed for the fourth time in eleven months, and this time a customer was also victimized. "My husband's been hit by a car, he's screaming. There's blood everywhere, and his left leg . . . oh my God. We need help!"

That lady in exam room A is speechless because this morning she was raped at gunpoint. There's a man in the school and he's shooting. An angry mob just entered the town square and cars are burning. We need help.

On April 8, 2020, the NYPD reported 132 new coronavirus cases in a 24-hour period. Sadly, 13 members of the NYPD had lost their lives due to complications from coronavirus. A total of 7,130 uniformed members were on sick leave as a result. Who would be next? They need help.

The officer's partner died last night, shot four times as he approached a routine traffic violation. Many officers are nervous on duty working in crowds and in large public gatherings. "I remember the boy's eyes. I remember the feces and garbage everywhere, the used syringes, the absence of electricity. The mother was not close to conscious. So vivid are the boy's eyes, I can't sleep." They need help.

The officer waved to a group of young teens on their bikes, but most gave him the middle finger. Last week he was spit at, doused with water, called a Pig, told to burn in hell. "A number of us have broken marriages, we got shrinks, we are scared our partners will eventually find out." How long can they take this? They need help.

Of course there are many sides to complex stories and situations. Of course there are good cops and bad. Of course there's corruption, bigotry, and misconduct. But America, think about "we need" and think about "they need."

To every man and woman who has ever worn a police uniform, I honor you, I respect you, and I thank you for your service from the bottom of my heart.

I see you standing in the emergency department late at night, in the trenches with the rest of us doing our best to serve others. I see you sitting in the hall guarding that patient's room, the teenager shot by a gang. I see the badge, the protective vest, the man or woman who wants to help our fallen world.

To all officers, we need your help. To all officers, and for those of you who need our help, thank you for serving.

Because They Have To

There are so many similarities among people who choose to serve as their profession. Physicians, APPs, nurses, teachers, military, firefighters, police officers, and many others. There's a common wiring, a common DNA, a calling that "I want to help others."

In a world of "it's all about me, it's all about money, it's all about winning and fame," servant leaders must serve first, and these others factors are at best secondary.

People who serve are different. They run toward danger, not from. They help people knowing that others may not help them. There's no expectation, there's no deal or quid pro quo. First responders place the needs of others before their own. And they do so because they have to. Serving others provides them strength, it powers their love, it defines their truth. It is their why.

Anything less is unacceptable—to their heart, to their soul, to their conscience. And when they stop serving, it can promote stress and burnout versus joy and fulfillment. But it's tough to keep giving when others take. Whether it's at work, in the community, or with personal relationships, it's a heavy cross to bear. It can be pretty discouraging and disappointing falling on your sword for others, especially when it's not appreciated or reciprocated.

It's tough for a teacher to keep loving teaching when students and parents are always right. It's tough for a nurse to care for patients when she was just belittled by one, again. It's tough to restart the squad car knowing you infected your kids with the coronavirus just weeks earlier. It's tough standing six feet apart on the USNS *Comfort* when you know that many Americans criticize the military. It's tough to accept that your scarred lungs from 9/11 won't last much longer, knowing that many in society never acknowledged firefighters prior to the disaster. Yes, it's tough to serve.

I just wish that more of us were better at appreciating and respecting those who serve. That we would place ourselves in their shoes and realize how difficult their calling is. I cry out to my fellow Americans for us to rethink how we treat one another, and especially those who serve our country daily.

Please remember the faces of the first responders. A thank you. A thumbs-up. Better still, a hug. That's all they need. So simple, but so life-giving to those who serve. To those who serve because they have to.

To all of you, with a fist pump, thank you for serving.

TEAM TALK

To my fellow nurses and APPs: thank you so much for joining me and other physicians as we all try to better equip ourselves to use our gifts and talents to help others and to serve, to fight burnout, and to find joy as healthcare providers. I am so proud of each and every one of you.

God bless you all. Cheers!

A JOURNEY MOMENT

I hope that *Fist Pumps* has been beneficial and encouraging. I have really enjoyed our journey together. Don't hesitate to reread some of the chapters over and over. Think. Write. Speak. And then live out your calling to serve others. Use the book as a starting point that will help take you on a magnificent journey to live on your mountaintop and to finish strong.

Before you close the book, I have one last journaling exercise that you must complete.

Raise up your dominant forearm with your fist clenched. Begin swinging it downward with a vigorous pumping motion. Look up to God or a higher power, or look inward for strength and encouragement and then say with me: "I've got this. I can do it. I was called to serve!"

Congratulations, you have now joined the Fist Pumps Revolution. You have been a wonderful student. I am so proud of you. Good luck on your journey to your mountaintop, and God bless.

CLIMB TO THE SUMMIT TOGETHER

By reading *Fist Pumps: The Prescription for Physician Burnout* you have officially joined the Fist Pumps Revolution. You have begun your journey to the mountaintop, and you are determined to be joyful and fulfilled as a physician and healthcare provider. The battle against burnout is a difficult journey, and we will be more successful when we climb to the summit together.

Yes, thousands of like-minded people can create a world that lifts up physicians and healthcare providers who serve. We can nourish and help one another, and as one voice we can make a significant impact. Visit fistpumpsrx.com and share any solutions and survival tactics that you have implemented or modified from reading *Fist Pumps*, or better still, add new ideas that you find beneficial.

There, please find the space where you can recommend other useful resources. Whether it's a book, a podcast, a YouTube video, a song, or something you learned from a colleague or friend, please share it with the Fist Pumps community and help make fistpumpsrx.com a tremendous resource. Don't underestimate the power of your words. You never know who you may rescue with your love and encouragement.

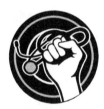

Download the Fist Pumps Revolution app. The app was designed to be your own personal cheerleader by counting your fist pumps and connecting you with others climbing to the summit. By officially joining the Fist Pumps Revolution and sharing encouraging and informative communications, we can support one another in our journeys.

Invite and urge others to join our journey and to share their experiences. It's time for us to create a world in which doctors love being doctors. One that nurses and advanced practice providers are excited and proud to care for our nation. Yes, it's time to start the Fist Pumps Revolution!

A Prayer

Dear God,

You gave healthcare providers gifts and talents to help others and to serve.

You designed us to heal the sick, to comfort the worried, and to sacrifice for others.

You hand-picked us, knowing that the health of the nation rests on our shoulders. It's an enormous responsibility. For many, it's a heavy cross to bear.

God, You know that many providers are struggling in the valley of burnout as they love and care for their patients. They are discouraged, angry, bitter, fearful, and others have lost hope.

Please reach out Your transcendent and loving hand to those in the valley and provide them the strength, the courage, and the peace to live their purpose, to live their why.

Please give each and every one of us the power of the Holy Spirit that will enable us to ascend to our mountaintop and to finish strong.

Without You, the journey is too difficult.

Amen.

ACKNOWLEDGMENTS

To my editor Betsy Thorpe:

Thank you, Betsy, for caring, for encouraging, and giving every ounce of your patience and excellence to my book. Thanks for allowing me to be Scott, to repeat myself, and for laughing at my jokes. Thanks for giving me your guidance, your beautiful voice, and most importantly, you! You are an incredible person who God has given so many talents. I will value our friendship forever. Cheers.

To Josh Landau, MD:

Josh, how do I begin to thank you for everything you have done for me? You provided me your time and strength when you were overwhelmed and weakened. You shared with me your gift of writing, your endless knowledge, your encouragement, and most of all, your caring for myself and for physicians nationwide. You have the mind, the strength, and most of all, the heart of a warrior. You are truly special.

Our friendship and journey may have started in an operating room locker room but it will finish on our mountaintop of joy and fulfillment. I cannot thank you enough for joining and helping me ascend to the summit, together. Fist pumps!

To Diana Wade:

Thank you, Diana, for putting together my labor of love. Your advice and insight was always appreciated. The book cover is phenomenal. I hope you had a wonderful trip to Nova Scotia. Thank you so much.

To Katherine Bartis:

Katherine, thank you for your copyediting and proofing and helping Betsy and I decorate the cake. The book is so much sweeter because of your valuable input.

To my friends and staff at Green Joe's Coffee Company:

Candy, thanks to you and the wonderful staff for your kindness and friendship. Sipping House Italian dark roast in "my spot" while writing *Fist Pumps* will be a memory I will treasure forever. Cheers!

Recommended Reading

Andrews, Andy. *The Traveler's Gift*. Nashville, TN: Thomas Nelson, 2002.

Covey, Stephen R. *The 7 Habits of Highly Effective People*. New York, NY: Simon & Schuster, 1989.

Drummond, Dike. *Stop Physician Burnout: What to Do When Working Harder Isn't Working*. Heritage Press Publications, 2014.

Warren, Rick. *The Purpose Driven Life*. Grand Rapids, MI: Zondervan, 2002.

ABOUT THE AUTHOR

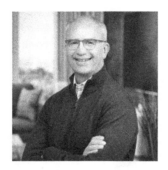

Dr. Scott MacDiarmid is deeply interested in and regularly speaks about healthcare and physician burnout. His lofty goal is to provide a world that lifts up physicians and other healthcare providers who serve. Dr. MacDiarmid is director of the Alliance Urology Specialists Bladder Control Center in Greensboro, NC. He completed fellowships in reconstructive urology and urodynamics at Duke University Medical Center in Durham, NC; the University of Otago in Christchurch, New Zealand; and the University of Sheffield in England. He is currently a clinical assistant professor of urology in the Department of Urology at the University of North Carolina in Chapel Hill, NC.

Printed in the USA
CPSIA information can be obtained
at www.ICGtesting.com
LVHW010701240923
758983LV00004B/16